When Does Human Life Begin?

When Does Human Life Begin?

Scientific, Scriptural, and Historical Evidence Supports Implantation

John L. Merritt, MD, FACP

J. Lawrence Merritt, II, MD

When Does Human Life Begin?

Scientific, Scriptural, and Historical Evidence Supports Implantation

by

John. L. Merritt, M.D., F.A.C.P.

J. Lawrence Merritt, II, M.D.

3rd Edition, published 2012 by

Crystal Clear Books

Kenmore, Washington, United States of America

Find us on the Web at:

http://www.LifeBeginsWhen.com

http://www.CrystalClearBooks.org

10 9 8 7 6 5 4 3 2 1

Table of Contents

Chapter 1   Introduction: When Human Life Begins   1

Chapter 2   Ancient and Christian History: In the Ancient Greek and Roman World   9

       In Christian History   14

Chapter 3   British and American Culture   27

       In America   29

Chapter 4   The Biology of Life's Beginning   33

       Mitosis   33

       Meiosis   34

       Imprinting   38

       Genetic Identity   40

       Blastocyst Viability—and Implantation   41

Chapter 5   The Biblical Evidence: The Breath of Life & Life in the Womb   45

       Breath of Life   47

       Life in The Womb … in Utero   50

Chapter 6   Blood … The Key   55

       Blood: The Missing Link in Life's First Breath   58

Chapter 7   A Compelling Case for Implantation   63

Notes and References: 67

Additional Resources   76

Chapter 1

Introduction:
When Human Life Begins

The Problem:

"Life begins at conception."

"A woman has a right to choose."

Choice ... Abortion ... but what about Life?

As we begin the second decade of the 21st century, one of history's greatest debates continues to passionately divide Americans and people worldwide. This dispute has been ongoing in hundreds of societies throughout recorded history. This book provides an in-depth review of that debate. More importantly, it offers a convincing solution that brings reason, clarity, and support through clear and compelling scientific, scriptural, and historical evidence. This evidence clearly demonstrates that human life begins, not at conception, but shortly after implantation of the *blastocyst* into a mother's uterus. This occurs on day eight after fertilization, when the mother's blood begins to provide the breath of life to the implanted blastocyst.

While abortion is the primary focus of this debate, arguments spill over into the areas of stem cell research and contraception. At the crux of these issues is the ultimate question:

When does human life begin?

The answers given are often nebulous—fraught with emotion, conflicting opinions, historical uncertainties, and general confusion. With all the information at our fingertips in today's digital age, from science, to scripture, to history, and to ethics, it is unfortunate and somewhat sad that we have continued in confusion. Although some have personal opinions based on political, theological, and social agendas, most have based their conclusions on what they have been told or personally deduced. Since there is such a massive and varied spectrum of information known, or unknown, some think it is natural that these seemingly never-ending varied positions should be acceptable in our pluralistic societies.

In contrast, we submit this state of confusion and indecision should not be accepted as conclusive. We, the authors of this book, contend that there is much information across a variety of disciplines that is generally overlooked and frequently not considered. A definitive conclusion is possible.

In fact, there is clear, and compelling, scientific and scriptural evidence that ***human life begins shortly after implantation of a blastocyst, on day eight after fertilization.***

Our scientific evidence focuses on the critical biology, genetics and epigenetics, and timing of implantation when the mother begins nourishing the blastocyst with her life supporting, replenishing blood.

The scriptural evidence is based on the God-given "breath of life," given to all as the cardinal definition of life as a living soul, a nephesh chaya (in Hebrew). But this breath of life is distributed by the blood and thus, the recurring theme of scripture is "the life is in the blood."

The following book chapters present a history of ancient and modern philosophies and examine how they have led to today's misconceptions regarding both pro-life and pro-choice political positions.

The understanding of human life's origin at implantation, when the life-giving blood of the mother first provides the "breath of life" to an implanted blastocyst—now a true embryo—now a "living soul"—will provide clarity and focus for evidenced-based deliberations in personal, social, political, and moral decision making.

We aspire to present this information in a way that encourages all—scientists, biologists, theologians, historians, educators, activists, politicians, and the general public—to reach an evidence-based, informed consensus regarding when human life *really* begins.

> **...there is, in fact, clear and compelling scientific, scriptural, and historical information that is generally overlooked and frequently not considered.**

By defining when human life begins, with clear and consistent evidence-based reasoning, we will provide a framework for personal and collective resolution of these often confusing and controversial issues.

The lack of a clear consensus, or even consistent reasoning, from experts in the theological, philosophical, political, and scientific communities is remarkable. In each of these communities there is wide diversity of opinion. A need for clarity is cited, but clarity remains absent. These disparate views are reliant on tradition and personal agendas, often with little scientific, historical, or ethical basis. Inflammatory language, misquotes of sources, and inconsistent terminology fan the flames of emotion and mistrust. This situation only complicates ethical and social policy decisions. Oliver recently (cynically, but truthfully) stated, "If life is only what we say it is, and begins only when we say it does, then we can say anything we like, and we will never be wrong."[1] As a result, there is a host of divergent opinions, quoting from historical practices, traditions, public health needs, political agendas, or scientific and medical promises in order to defend their conflicting positions.

> **The continuing lack of consensus from experts in the theological, philosophical, political, and scientific communities is remarkable.**

Various groups have also used specific time points in the biology of human development to distinguish and defend their idea of when life actually begins. They highlight a variety of different embryological events, such as: *gastrulation* (formation of the germ layers), first heartbeat, the *quickening* (first notable movement), recognizable human body shape, *neurulation* (the first appearance of a nervous system), and first brain waves. Other clinical time points include: *viability* (when the fetus could survive outside the womb), birth (delivery from the uterus), the first

3

breath of air, and finally to specific time marks following delivery at 40 days, 80 days, 90 days, 120 days, 15 weeks, 28 weeks, 3 months, 6 months, and 9 months. Table 1 provides a summary list of these and other various proposed events (or biological "landmarks") throughout history, beginning with conception (fusion of the sperm and ova).

Table 1: Historical Developmental Milestones Proposed as the Beginning of Life.	
Conception – sperm-ova union	
Zygote – single cell stage	
Mitosis – two cells in 12 hrs; into four cells in 24 hrs	
Morula – 16 or more cells	
Functional genotype development, methylation	
Blastocyst – inner cell separation and continuing division	
Blastocyst – adherence to uterine endothelium	
Implantation of blastocyst	
Reciprocal chemical exchanges between embryo and mother	
Blood interaction of hormones and nourishment	
Gastrulation – appearance of primitive streak	
Separation into embryonic germ layers	
First heart beat	
Vital organ development	
First brain waves	
Human form characteristics – eye, limb development	
Quickening – maternal detection of fetal movement	
Viability, with technologies	
Viability, without technological support	
Birth, first breath of air following delivery	
Nursing of the newborn infant	
Circumcision of the male infant	@8 days following birth
Naming of the infant	@8-40 days, 3-6 months
Weaning of the infant	@6-9 months

The argument over when life begins includes an interesting array of contributors. On one side, there are conservative authorities such as the Pope; the Roman Catholic Church; Christian fundamentalists and the evangelical right; social conservatives, most Republicans; many Democrats; many Hindu and Buddhist followers; and the orthodox Jewish community. Together they advocate for a legal position that life starts at fertilization (called conception in humans, the union of the sperm

4

and egg). This position imposes many implications on abortion, stem-cell research, and contraception issues. The fertilized human egg, before implantation into the mother's uterus, is called a *zygote*. The advocacy of a human life beginning at conception is referred to as the *personhood of the zygote*.[2, 3, 4] As conservative voices continue to rise, and claim a scriptural foundation for their fervor, they offer no clear and compelling scriptural evidence in support of life beginning at conception or for the personhood of the zygote. Texts used are usually broad and non-specific, requiring *eisegesis* (reading one's opinion into the text).

> **Ethicists refer to advocacy of a human life beginning at conception as *the personhood of the zygote*.**

On the other side, abortion rights advocates include many traditional Protestant communities, liberal Catholics, some moderate Republicans, the majority of Democrats, feminists, the political progressive left, most Conservative and Reformed Jews, most Muslims, secular humanists, the non-religious, the American Civil Liberties Union, and the Supreme Court.[5, 6, 7, 8, 9, 10, 11, 12, 13, 14]

In fact, the U.S. Supreme Court ruled on abortion in 1973, establishing a precedent for future rulings in lower U.S. courts. But the Court, in so doing, deliberately sidestepped the question as to when human life begins. The product of this omission was a decision, regarding abortion restrictions, in the landmark Roe vs. Wade case resulting in an arbitrary and consequent legal opinion that a fetus' life and value must, for practical purposes, reach "a compelling point." This point would be that of viability—when the fetus could survive outside the mother's womb, but the Court did not specifically state when such a point actually occurs (additional details follow in Chapter 3).[15, 16, 17, 42]

> **The U.S. Supreme Court deliberately sidestepped the question as to when human life begins.**

The Roe vs. Wade decision drew the first line in the sand as the end of the first trimester (12 weeks). This is still surprising, since in 1973 viability was from 24 to 28 weeks, based on the capabilities of medical care and technology in 1973. The decision gave individual states the authority to restrict abortion after the first trimester, but left guidelines for allowing abortion after that point if the continued pregnancy would endanger the mother's life or health. Significantly, this included her emotional and social health.[17, 18]

Other 20th century attempts to provide a scientific basis for political and social decisions were not limited to the controversial U.S. Supreme Court. Addressing not abortion, but embryonic research, across the Atlantic the government of Great Britain charged the Warnock Committee with setting up rules to regulate such research.[18, 36, 43]

> **In Great Britain the Warnock Committee adopted a policy that human life begins 14 days after fertilization, a time called gastrulation, when the "primitive streak," the precursor to the central nervous system, appeared.**

The Committee scientifically addressed the question of when human life begins. After much input and deliberation, the Committee adopted a policy that human life begins 14 days after fertilization, a time called gastrulation, when the *primitive streak* (the precursor to the central nervous system) appeared. The reason for selecting this time was that after gastrulation, spontaneous division of the blastocyst to form twins (known as twinning) was not possible. The Commission reasoned that the embryo, after gastrulation, might unequivocally be termed an individual, not a twin. Thus an individual, a person, existed at this point, and consequentially a sacrifice of the embryo for scientific research should be limited. One may conclude, that on the surface, this reasoning may be attractive. Similarly, few could argue that the Warnock Committee in Great Britain had a much more firm scientific foundation than the U.S. Supreme Court's "practical" compromise, although its focus was not on abortion, but on fetal cell and stem cell research and is much less well known.[17, 41]

The inability to arrive at a definitive consensus to such an important question has recently been underlined by the publication of a report by the President's Council on Bioethics in 2008.

> **The President's Council on Bioethics in 2008 called for a deeper understanding of the foundations upon which we build our answers to life's most challenging questions**

In the commissioned volume, including an address to the President, the Council stated, "These essays make it clear that there is no universal agreement on the meaning of the term, human dignity." But then reported that, "An appreciation of the variety of these views is critical...." The Council then called for "a deeper understanding of the foundations upon which we build our answers to life's most challenging questions."

This book, we submit, will present important and compelling evidence that has not been regarded or reported, that when considered, will provide fundamental answers to this most challenging question: *When does human life begin?*

> **We will in this book answer that question, by presenting compelling evidence that human life begins shortly after implantation of a blastocyst, on day eight after fertilization, when a mother's blood first gives the "breath of life" to the new human life, thus becoming a "living soul."**

7

Chapter 2

Ancient and Christian History:
In the Ancient Greek and Roman World

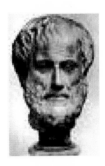

Diversity of opinion about when human life begins is not new.

The debate extends into the very roots of western civilization, that of ancient Greece. Greek culture contributed lasting patterns to Western culture including democracy, science, mathematics, art, literature, logic, and religion. A key to Greek culture, in all these areas, was their thoughts about beauty and form. They idealized the human body, its proportions, and its form. Affecting their literature, everyday lives, religion, and science, the ancient Greek's idealization of form extended beyond their arts and athletics.

Early Greek civilization, however, like most western civilizations, was not homogeneous. Several schools of philosophy developed. Each school, although a rival of the others, contributed to lasting western philosophical concepts in culture, law, science, and religion. The Pythagoreans were a mystical school, and are most well known today for their Pythagorean theorem, a key mathematical relationship in geometry and trigonometry. The Pythagoreans were introspective about the meaning of life, the substance of an individual, and his relationship to nature. They stressed the concept of a *soul* as the essence of an individual's existence.[17] They reasoned that a human soul was created at the time of conception. This is the earliest record of the concept that remains so prevalent today.

The Greek system produced many famous early physicians, starting with Aesculapius. Aesculapius was perhaps a real person, but was worshipped as the god of medicine, and said to be a son of Apollo and the daughter of a human king. His school of medicine left a lasting imprint on modern medicine with its staff of Aesculapius, a snake wrapped around a wooden rod. The version with two snakes and wings positioned at the top, often published today, is actually a symbol of Mercury, not Aesculapius.

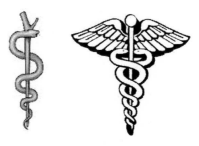

Hippocrates, the world's most famous physician and traditional father of medicine, was said to be the 15th generation descendant of Aesculapius. The medical-philosophy-temple cult of Aesculapius-Hippocrates adhered to Pythagorean concepts relating to the soul. This reasoning is reflected in the famous Hippocratic Oath, which is still with us today in the 21st century CE. However, it represented a minority position in ancient BCE Greece society, where abortion and infanticide was commonly practiced.[18] The Oath did ban abortion by Aesculapian-Hippocratic trained physicians. It also expressly forbade giving a woman "an instrument to produce abortion." This is interpreted as forbidding abortion by any method. Hippocrates' disapproval of abortion stemmed from his belief that conception marked the beginning of human life, as taught by the Pythagoreans and the Aesculapian temple cult.

> **The famous Hippocratic Oath was based on the Pythagorean belief that the soul began at conception, and it expressly forbade giving a woman "an instrument to produce abortion."**

Two other Greek concepts about the human soul—*delayed ensoulment* and *animation*—have had even more influence on religious and secular opinions over the ages. The most influential Greek school of philosophy was the Socrates-Plato-Aristotle school. Socrates trained Plato, who then trained Aristotle, who was the tutor of Alexander the Great. They lived in the golden age of Greek culture, the 5th–4th centuries BCE. After Alexander the Great conquered much of the civilized world, Greek, or *Hellenistic*, thought and culture prevailed over western civilization. The Greek rationalistic beliefs of Socrates-Plato-Aristotle dominated this wave of Hellenistic thought, which spread throughout the world—continuing through thousands of years into the thoughts of our present "modern" age.

> **Plato taught that a human soul does not enter the body until birth, and abortion should be compelled in any woman after age 40. Although sexual intercourse is permitted after 40, every effort should be made to prevent children conceived from seeing light, to dispose of the newborn child if necessary.**

Much can be discussed about the many aspects of this system of philosophy, but we will focus on their concepts relating to human life, the human soul, when a human life begins, and abortion. In later chapters, we will explore the effects of these concepts in modern society, science, religion and politics, while offering a compelling evidence-based alternative.

Plato proposed his ideal worldview in "The Republic," his still famous version of utopia. In this ideal world, he addressed the most prevalent Greek view of the soul. He defended a position, based on the ideal of perfect form, that the human soul does not enter the body until birth. This greatly influenced legal science in Greece, and subsequently extended down the centuries into the Roman Empire and then the Middle Ages.

11

> **Aristotle described the concept of *delayed ensoulment* and *animation*, with evolution from an unformed "vegetable soul" to a formed "animal soul" then finally into a "human soul".**

In "The Republic," Plato wrote that abortion should be compelled in any woman who becomes pregnant after 40. Plato's Republic made eugenics a matter of policy in a utopian society—a policy that parents should bear children for the state, and for only a defined period of years. After that period, sexual intercourse would be permitted, but the couple involved would make every effort to prevent any children conceived from "seeing light" (i.e., being born alive). The policy stated that when this was not possible, they were to dispose of the newborn child.[17, 19]

Aristotle expanded on, and further elucidated, extant views about the human soul. His logic was first widely articulated in about 350 BCE. Aristotle described the concepts of delayed ensoulment and animation. Building upon the classical Greek appreciation and elevation of form in nature and life, he taught that a fetus was, at first, an unformed "vegetable soul". This evolved into an "animal soul" later in gestation. It finally became "animated" with a formed human soul.[17, 18, 44] This was the process of *ensoulment*. Fetal ensoulment was reasoned by the early Greeks to be at 40 days for male, and 90 days for females (a non-distinction, though, in reality since the ability to determine fetal sex *in utero* was still millennia away, and remains difficult even today prior to 12 weeks gestation). These concepts dominated western classical thought over the next 600 years.

Aristotle's teachings powerfully influenced and helped formulate western history's most persistent view on abortion and the beginning of human life. As we discussed earlier, his concept of delayed ensoulment with its reasoned support of abortion was widely accepted. It was also applied to politics. Aristotle believed the state should fix the number of children a married couple could have (note the similarity to modern Communist China's policies). While Aristotle held the common Greek view that deformed children ought not to be reared, he objected to the abandonment of healthy infants merely as a method of population control. In his view, if children were conceived in excess of the permitted number, an abortion should be procured at an early stage of pregnancy "before sensation and life develop in the embryo."[17, 19, 27]

In Aristotle's opinion, delayed ensoulment occurred on the 40th day after conception in the case of a male child and on the 90th day for a female.

Aristotle went further and detailed the notion of the animation of the fetus, where individuality, life, and form were features for which the soul was responsible at certain points of gestation. Aristotle asserted that when a soul was added to the amorphous matter in the womb, a living individuated creature was created, which had the potential for form and the rational power of a man. The movement of the fetus in the womb reflected this process of formation, or animation. Aristotle's opinion was similar to other early Greeks, stating this took place at 40 or 90 days after conception for male or female children, respectively. Aristotle explained this difference in animation times was based on what he perceived to be fundamental differences between men and women. Aristotle believed that males were more active than females, thus males were quicker to develop, obtain a soul, and become animated within the womb. Females, on the other hand, were viewed as physically and intellectually inferior to men. This logic led to the conclusion that the female process of ensoulment would take longer to complete.

Aristotle advocated state control of birth rate. If children were conceived in excess of the permitted number, an abortion should be procured at an early stage of pregnancy "before sensation and life develop in the embryo".

Another somewhat less influential, yet very strict Greek school of philosophy was the Stoics. They believed the fetus was no more than a part or extension of the women's body during the entire duration of pregnancy. They taught that ensoulment occurred only at birth, when cooling by the air transformed a lump of flesh into a living and sentient being.

At times, the distinction as to when human life begins was based not on philosophy or ethics, but on a community's perceived need to regulate its population size. In another ancient Greek society, Sparta, abortion was frowned upon because it ran counter to the desire to raise strong males for military struggles. Yet, the practice of leaving a child to die of

13

exposure on a hillside was not considered murder if the child was judged to be unsuitable for some reason. It is unclear whether Spartans believed if one obtained personhood after birth, and the regulation on abortion was purely for political reasons, or if they believed personhood was obtained prior to birth, and it was a status unattainable by deformed infants.

The Hellenistic views of Plato and Aristotle set the tone for the following empire—Rome. In fact, the Romans considered the Greek and Roman religions to be one and the same, and one of the four official religions of the early Roman Empire. Greek philosophy was inherent in the Roman way of life, although the Romans were somewhat less philosophical and more bent on the practical. The ancient Romans did not openly approve or advocate the practice of abortion, but it was not considered a serious offense, and was not regulated. Indeed, a leading Roman historian named Seneca disapprovingly reported that it was common practice for a woman to induce abortion in order to maintain the beauty of her figure.[17]

This background of ancient history gives us a foundation to better understand the world as early Christian teachings were developed.

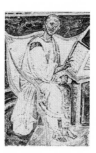

In Christian History

The Romans accepted only four religions *officially* within their territories:

- The Greek-Roman state religion
- The Egyptian state religion
- Judaism

- Mithraism

But in the middle of the 1ˢᵗ century CE, another religion was rapidly spreading through its territories—Christianity. Initially considered a sect of Judaism, its evangelism brought conflict with the official Roman religions and law. Christianity quickly spread, even while splitting into competing groups. Each was fiercely evangelical, with a prime directive to "go into the whole world and make disciples of all men." By the end of the 1ˢᵗ century CE, there were three major and competing branches within this new religion:

- Orthodox (Catholic)
- Jewish Christianity (variously: Nazarene, Ebionite, Messianic)
- Gnostic

Of these three branches of Christianity, only the Orthodox (Catholic) form survived and flourished into the 4ᵗʰ century CE. At that time the emperor himself, Constantine, accepted Christianity. He soon made it another official religion of the empire, and in time, THE official religion. This Rome-based Christianity became the model for Western Christianity that is practiced by the majority of Christians today. When the young and rapidly expanding Orthodox (Roman-Catholic) Christianity became the official state religion of the Roman Empire in 312 CE, it was still surrounded by competing religions:

The official old four:

- The Greek-Roman state religion
- The Egyptian religion
- Rabbinical Judaism
- Mithraism

And now completing versions of Christianity:

- Gnosticism
- Jewish Messianic Christianity (Nazarenes, Ebionites, Elkesaites, etc, by now already declining in numbers)

With the exception of Judaism, all of the old pagan religions had allowed women to have abortions. They also allowed parents to strangle or expose (abandon) newborn babies as methods of population control. But Judaism and its offshoot Christian branches were initially opposed to abortion. The ever-present, long held Hellenistic ideas of the Greeks and Romans, however, would over time influence the development of Orthodox Christian thought about when life begins, and would impact the Church's positions on abortion.

During the first three centuries C.E, while Christianity was spreading thru a pagan world, abortion was the norm (as we discussed in the previous chapter). As Christianity was primarily based on its Jewish roots, all of the early forms of Christianity mirrored early Judaism. The earliest Christian philosophers and Fathers (100–300 CE) equated abortion with infanticide and condemned both as murder.[20, 44]

> **With the exception of the two forms of Judaism, all of early Christianity's competitors allowed women to have abortions, and even encouraged parents to strangle or expose (abandon) newborn babies as methods of population control.**

Among the earliest Christian manuscripts in existence are the Didache (reflections of early 2nd century primitive Christian believers), the works of Barnabas, and the Apocalypse of Peter. All three of these documents condemned abortion.[20, 21, 22, 23]

The Didache says, "You shall not murder a child by abortion." The writings and teachings of many early Church Fathers reflected the same prohibition during the first centuries of Christian development.

> **On abortion, the early opinions of Christianity mirrored the two major forms of first century Judaism: Rabbinical and Jewish Messianic Christianity. Both were distinctly anti-abortion.**

Tertullian, an early and prominent Christian theologian, wrote extensively on abortion, among other topics. He opposed abortion, early and late, as well as contraception. He regarded them as "proleptic murder"—the prevention of a birth that should occur.[24]

In his Apology (CE. 197) Tertullian denounces infanticide and abortion:

"As regards infanticide, however—although I grant that murder of a child, if it is your own, differs from killing somebody else! It makes no difference whether it is done willfully or as part of a sacred rite. I will turn to you now as a nation. How many of the crowd standing round us, open-mouthed for Christian blood, how many of you, gentlemen, magistrates most just and strict against us, shall I not prick in your inner consciousness as being the slayers of your own offspring? There is, indeed, a difference in the manner of death; but assuredly it is crueler to drown an infant or expose it to cold and starvation and the dogs (than to sacrifice it, as you allege that we do) even an adult would prefer to die by the sword. But for us, to whom homicide has been once for all forbidden, it is not permitted to break up even what has been conceived in the womb, while the blood is still being drawn from the mother's body to make a new creature. Prevention of birth is premature murder, and it makes no difference whether it is a life already born that one snatches away or a life that is coming to birth that one destroys. The future of man is a man already: the whole fruit is present in the seed." [25]

Tertullian observes that infanticide, usually accomplished by exposure, was generally accepted in 2nd century CE Roman society. He contends it was only eventually banned due to the influence of Christianity. He is quite likely right. The notion that a child, once born, was a human being enjoying the same right to life as an adult was very far from acceptance by Roman society. The survival of the child during the first few days following birth depended to a great degree upon the decision of the father, who thus retained the power of life and death enjoyed by the head of the family in Roman society. This residual patriarchal power perished with the instillation of Christianity; but the notion that parents had a right over the fate of the newly born was retained.

> **Tertullian said, "But for us, to whom homicide has been forbidden, it is not permitted to break up even what has been conceived in the womb, while the blood is still being drawn from the mother's body to make a new creature."**

While Tertullian regarded infanticide and abortion as forms of homicide, indicating he believed the fetus had acquired a status of humanness, he did recognize the need for abortions when necessary to save the life of the mother. St. Basil the Great, Bishop of Caesarea, was considered one of early Christianity's foremost scholars. In CE 374, he reinforced Tertullian's views when he also declared that abortion was murder and no distinction between the formed and the unformed fetus was admissible in Christian morality.[17]

Over the centuries, however, Hellenistic doctrines, directly from the teachings of Aristotle and Plato, became increasingly influential among Christian scholars and leaders. These writings greatly affected St. Augustine, who, by the end of the 4th century CE, became the most prolific and influential writer of the early Christian church fathers.

In 400 CE, St. Augustine wrote that a human soul could not live in an unformed body (using classical Greek reasoning, with emphasis on its visual "form"). He agreed with Aristotle's concept of delayed ensoulment. Augustine stated that in early pregnancy, an abortion is not murder since no soul is destroyed, or more accurately stated, only a vegetable or animal soul is terminated.[17, 26, 27] He concluded that only the abortion of a fully developed "fetus animatus"—an animated fetus—was murder.

> **Over the centuries, however, and by the time of St. Augustine, the Aristotle-Hellenistic influences became more influential in Christianity.**

The other famous 5th century CE church scholar was St. Jerome. His extensive writings are still widely used, and it was he who translated the entire Bible into Latin. Writing around the same time, Jerome concurred with Augustine in his letter to Aglasia that: "The seed gradually takes shape in the uterus, and it (abortion) does not count as killing until the individual elements have acquired their external appearance and their limbs."[28] This position continued to be the dominant and most widely accepted view of the beginning of human life, and reflected on the Western Church's view on abortion, for the next fourteen centuries.

The Eastern Orthodox Church broke with the Roman Catholic Church on a number of issues and was generally less influenced by Hellenism and the Latin fathers. The various Orthodox churches, such as the Greek,

Russian, Ukrainian, Coptic, Macedonian, and Assyrian, were more consistent in adhering to a tradition against abortion. To this day, they have generally held to the position that human life begins at conception. The Roman Catholic Church, however, wavered over time regarding the issue of when human life begins; wavering more than is widely known to the public, to parishioners, and more than is admitted by the Vatican.

> **In 400 CE, St. Augustine wrote "a human soul could NOT live in an unformed body" using classical Greek reasoning, with emphasis on its visual form. He concurred with, and articulated the teachings of, Aristotle: the concept of delayed ensoulment.**

By the 5th century CE, other Catholic fathers, including St. Thomas Aquinas and St. Augustine of Hippo, joined Augustine and Jerome. They all adopted Aristotle's view that the fetus was animated (i.e., ensouled) around day 40.[40] This opinion was based on Hellenistic philosophy, and distinctly varied from the position of the early Jewish Nazarenes and the earliest Christian churches. The Hellenistic influences advocated by Augustine, Jerome, and these others dominated Roman Catholic teachings for 1400 years.

> **Jerome wrote, "The seed gradually takes shape in the uterus, and it (abortion) does not count as killing until the individual elements have acquired their external appearance and their limbs."**

Aristotle and Greek philosophy influenced early medieval Christian interpretations on abortion, and thus their views on when human life begins. This influence was also promoted via Greek translations of the writings in the Old Testament, with the most well known being the translation of the Hebrew Torah into a Greek text called the Septuagint. This subsequently included the entire Tanach: the Old Testament.

The Greek Septuagint versions of Exodus 21:22-23 included a distinction between an unformed and a formed fetus. The formed fetus was considered an independent person, while the unformed fetus was not.

Thus, a Greek-based Christian tradition was derived that disputed the earlier Hebrew-Jewish view. This stemmed from a mistranslation of a Hebrew term into the Greek in the Septuagint. The Hebrew word for "no harm follow" was replaced with the Greek word for "imperfectly formed".[22, 24, 28, 29]

The translation from the Greek Septuagint Exodus 21:23 is thus:

> "And if two men strive together and smite a woman with child, and her child be born *imperfectly formed*, he shall be forced to pay a penalty: as the woman's husband shall lay upon him he shall pay with valuation. But if it be *perfectly formed*, he shall give life for life." (Exodus 21:21-23).

> **By the 5th century CE, Augustine and Jerome and other Catholic fathers, including Thomas Aquinas and Augustine of Hippo, had all adopted Aristotle's view that fetuses were animated (ensouled) around day 40.**

The major church fathers accepted this interpretation, distinguishing between an unformed and a formed fetus, and branding only the killing of a formed fetus as murder. This provided a scriptural basis for the Aristotle-Hellenistic concept of delayed ensoulment. The formed fetus was to be accorded full human status.[12, 25] This distinction was subsequently embodied in canon law (official legal rulings by the Vatican) and later into Justinian's Law. Justinian, the Roman emperor, made Roman Catholic canon law the official Law of the Roman Empire, including the concepts of delayed ensoulment and animation.

> **Delayed ensoulment continued to be the accepted view of the beginning of human life, and reflected on the Western Church's view on abortion for the next 14 centuries.**

This presumed distinction between a formed and an unformed fetus, in the Greek version of Exodus, generated a question as to whether biblical writers understood embryonic development, and had designated a time point that marked the formation of a fetus.

20

The Tanach (Old Testament) does include several passages in which the growth of the unborn child is described. These verses are, however, written in poetry, and it cannot be determined whether they represent what the biblical writers actually thought was happening inside the womb.

Two examples of this are illustrated:

First we examine Job 10:10. Here Job states the rhetorical question.

> "Did you not pour me out like milk and curdle me like cheese?" Job continues, "You clothed me with skin and flesh, and knit me together with bones and sinews."

This reference to curdling may reflect the fact that as a result of miscarriages and premature births, the biblical writers were aware of the difference between the fetus in an undeveloped state, and in a state where the outward form of the child was already complete.

Early medieval Christian interpretations on abortion and when human life begins were influenced by Aristotle and Greek philosophy, and subsequently by Greek mistranslations from the original Hebrew Old Testament.

Next we see the author of Psalms explaining the growth of a child from formless, to developed and complete.

> "You formed my inward parts; you knitted me together in my mother's womb. I praise you, for I am fearfully and wonderfully made. Wonderful are your works; my soul knows it very well. My frame was not hidden from you, when I was being made in secret, intricately woven in the depths of the earth. Your eyes saw my unformed substance; in your book were written, every one of them, the days that were formed for me, when as yet there was none of them." (Psalms 139: 13-16)

Even though there is not a clear distinction indicating when a fetal body obtains a human form, and whether human form designates acquisition of humanness, there is a clear reference to the involvement of God in the process of growth and development of the embryo. Some modern day theologians, however, argue that there is no need to distinguish between unformed and formed fetal states, because embryonic development in vivo is a continuing divine process.

> **Gratian concluded "abortion was homicide only when the fetus was formed." If the fetus was not yet a formed human being, abortion was not homicide.**

Throughout history, we see that the Roman Catholic Church has held varying declarations about the beginning of human life. Actually, for most of the history of the Catholic Church, its thinkers viewed immediate animation/ensoulment as impossible. Under the traditional Catholic doctrine, a male fetus became animated—infused with a soul—at 40 days after conception, and the female fetus became animated at 80 days after conception.

Johannes Gratian, a 10th century CE Italian Catholic monk and scholar, is known as the founder of the science of canon law. He published the Concordantia discordantium canonum, generally called the Decretum Gratiani today. This first collection of canon law completed in 1140 CE was accepted as authoritative within the church. Among the many subjects he recorded, he included the current canon law on abortion. He concluded, "abortion was homicide only when the fetus was formed." If the fetus was not yet a formed human being, abortion was not homicide.

As late as 1261 CE, Pope Innocent III wrote a letter ruling on the case of a Carthusian monk who had arranged for his female lover to obtain an abortion. The Pope decided, consistent with canon law, that the monk was not guilty of homicide if the fetus was not animated. Pope Innocent III stated that the soul enters the body of the fetus at the time of quickening—when the woman first feels movement of the fetus. He ruled that after ensoulment, abortion was murder, but before ensoulment, abortion was a less serious sin, since it terminated only potential human life, not an actual human life.

In 1588 CE, however, Pope Sixtus V countered these laws. (This was Sixtus V, not Sixtus IV—for whom the Sistine Chapel was named.) Pope Sixtus V mandated that the penalty for abortion (and for contraception) to be excommunication from the Church. His successor, Pope Gregory IX, however, quickly returned the Church to the Hellenistic-Aristotle-

Augustinian view that abortion of an unformed embryo was not homicide. This demonstrates how discussion, debate and disagreements were continuing despite the official Catholic positions.[17, 33]

Official Catholic doctrine, firmly enunciated by Saint Augustine and other early Christian authorities, had also concluded that the unborn child was included among those condemned to eternal perdition if he died unbaptized. This was problematic in practice. A movement to remove the distinction between animate and inanimate fetuses from the Catholic doctrine was initiated by Thomas Fienus, an eminent physician and professor of medicine at Antwerp, and founder of hypnosis treatment methods. Dr. Fienus argued as early as 1620 that the soul must be present immediately after conception in order to organize the material of the body. Although his insights were only theoretical, lacking specific scientific methodology to study the biology of the events of the first few weeks in the womb, his insights were influential in the developing Catholic, Reformed, and Protestant thoughts.

In the late 19th century, following the scientific discovery and biological description of fertilization, the debate about abortion within the church shifted, again. It began to favor its now familiar position that human life begins at conception. An additional problematic issue was forced by the theological acceptance of the Immaculate Conception of Mary. In 1701 Pope Clement XI had declared the Immaculate Conception a feast of universal obligation.

Pope Pius IX served in the mid 19th century and became one of the most influential popes of the last two centuries. He instituted numerous lasting Papal decrees and theological updates. In 1854 Pope Pius IX incorporated into Catholic dogma the teaching that Mary was without sin from the moment of her conception. However, this did not coincide with the prior view that the fetus did not acquire a soul until later in pregnancy. So the church had to readdress its doctrine, making the act of conception the beginning of human life.

> **In 1869 Pope Pius IX officially reversed this long-held position on delayed ensoulment. He declared that the punishment for abortion (early and late) was to be excommunication. He concluded that since we cannot know with certainty the time at which human life begins, potential life should have protection from the earliest possible time, that of conception.**

The year 1869 was a bell-weather moment in Catholic and Christian history,[17] one that spills over into many other Christian bodies and into many national laws in the western world. The position of delayed ensoulment, long the official view of the Vatican, was overturned in 1869, when Pope Pius IX definitively declared that the punishment for abortion (early and late) was to be excommunication.

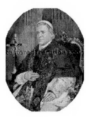

He considered the issues and finally concluded that since we do not and cannot know with certainty the time at which human life begins, potential life should have protection from the earliest possible time, that of conception. We should be clear that in this declaration, Pope Pius IX's view does not actually insist that fertilization is the time when human life begins. Rather, it is a statement that we do not and cannot know the time of ensoulment, therefore the most conservative position possible, i.e. conception, should be observed to save a life.

Pope Pius IX was also responsible for the canonization of Mary, with the declaration that Mary was born without sin. Her miraculous, sinless beginning was defined at her conception. This doctrine linked her beginning, and therefore human beginning, with conception.[34]

This principle is extremely important in defining present day Catholic doctrine relating to the "When does life begin?" question. The canonization of Mary and Immaculate Conception theology was a key link to Pope Pius IX's later declaration about abortion. In this context, his decision is natural and quite logical. If Mary's life began with her Immaculate Conception—there was no delayed ensoulment. So if there was no delayed ensoulment—then life begins at conception. Then for Mary, and all other human beings, any termination of the conceptus (a fetus) must be abortion.

This brings us to the current Roman Catholic Church doctrine maintained over the last 140 years—the belief in *immediate animation*—the instant in which the zygote is endowed with life, including a soul from God.[52] This "moment" is considered concurrent with the moment of fertilization. Catholic theologians over the last century and half have argued that the rational human soul also began at the time of conception, because such an infusion was considered a divine act. This designation established that ensoulment occurred at conception, and the zygote-blastocyst-fetus should be designated a status independent of its parents. The fetus was considered a separate entity, no longer an automatic derivative of its parents. Hence, it had now obtained a status of humanness as early as conception - a real and literal personhood of the zygote.[55, 56, 65]

Some Catholic theologians today carry this idea to its logical conclusion: they reject medical reasons for abortion. They consider abortion of an ova-sperm union as the destruction of a potential human being, and an outright refusal of a divine gift from God. This current Catholic viewpoint, however, strays from that of Jerome and Augustine, who accepted the use of abortion when the mother's life was threatened, countering the Church's current view that "two deaths are better than one murder." [22, 29]

To be fair and accurate, Catholicism has always discouraged abortion, even early abortion, in that it has long held that these acts interfered with the procreative purpose of sexual activity. But as we can see from the history documented above, for 1400 years the Church held that a fetus was not considered a person early in pregnancy, and early abortion was not deemed homicide, but a lesser violation.[17]

So the Roman Catholic Church's very influential belief that life begins at conception has evolved into a well-entrenched and now unwavering doctrine maintained to the present day. This belief assumes that potential life, even in the earliest stages of gestation, enjoys the same value as any existing life. The Catholic position has been adopted by a vast majority of Protestants, especially evangelical, fundamentalist, and charismatic Christians, and many other politically conservative Americans. We should note that the position of many Orthodox Jews is also anti-abortion, but for different Torah-based and Halacha reasons.[24, 28, 29]

In the experience of the authors, we have found the advocates of conception-life origin often lack supportive references when asked for scientific or scriptural evidence for life beginning at conception.. These advocates frequently cite seemingly simple and obvious emotional and traditional reasons, without fully understanding the complexity of the issue. The ultimate goal of this book is to provide a compelling look at what scripture and science *really* reveal about the subject matter.

> **The doctrine of the Immaculate Conception is that Mary, the mother of Jesus, was born without sin. Her miraculous beginning was defined at her conception.**

For even more historical detail and discussions, we would refer the reader to the comprehensive reviews in Gilbert, Tyler, Zackin's "Bioethics and The New Embryology" and in Gilbert, "Bioethics: When Does Life Begin?" and in Tribe, "Abortion: The Clash of the Absolutes."[17, 35, 36]

Chapter 3

British and American Culture

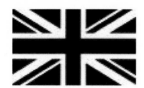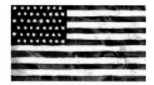

Originally, the abortion laws in Britain roughly coincided with medieval Catholic beliefs on when human life begins. But gradually, the multifaceted political aspects of abortion resulted in abortion laws deviating from general medieval opinion.

English common law initially saw the beginning of a human soul at quickening—believed to be the stage when the soul enters the body and the embryo could be felt moving within the uterus. This was consistent with Catholic theology and Aristotle-Hellenistic thought and believed to occur at about four months post-conception.

Abortion laws became more stringent in 1803, when abortion was criminalized. Punishment for abortion before quickening was exile, whipping, or imprisonment and post-quickening abortion could be punishable with death. In 1838, the concept of quickening was removed from the British legal rulings on abortion. At the same time, punishment by death was also eliminated. Under the Offenses Against the Person Act of 1861, anyone procuring an unlawful abortion, including the woman herself, could be punished with up to three years in prison.

In 1929 Parliament passed the Infant Life (Preservation) Act. This Act stated that a termination of pregnancy, particularly with a viable fetus, is unlawful except, when proven it was done in good faith, to preserve the life of the mother.[17]

> **English common law originally saw the beginning of a human soul at quickening.**

In 1966, the House of Commons voted to legalize abortions performed for medical reasons, including health. The British Abortion Act of 1967 permitted abortion until infant viability (when a delivered fetus could survive outside the womb). However, two doctors were required to certify that the risk to the life, mental or physical health of the woman, or to her existing children, would be greater if the pregnancy were to continue, than if it were to be terminated. But anti-abortion scholars have argued against the ethics of such a provision. A leading opponent being the Orthodox Chief Rabbi of the United Kingdom, Sir Immanuel Jacokovits.[28, 29]

The Infant Life Preservation Act to this day serves as a basis for defining a possible starting moment for life as the time of viability. This has been interpreted to restrict abortion after 28 weeks of gestational age, but viability depends on the use of technology and advances in technology. It is a paradox that as technology advances, making fetuses viable earlier, the legal allowance for abortion moves in the other direction. The Infant Life Preservation Act, though, is a legal definition—ambiguous and without sound scientific or ethical foundations. This kind of vague science and ethics has challenged the authors of this volume to explore the evidence and produce this report.

> **There is a paradox between technological advancement, which improves fetal viability after premature delivery, and the legal allowance for abortion, which moves in the opposite direction.**

More currently, the advancement of our medical and scientific knowledge has expanded the abortion debate to include stem cell research in the question of when does life begin. To address this challenging issue in Great Britain, the Warnock Committee was charged to set up rules to govern embryonic research. The Committee considered numerous gestational landmarks (see our review of potential landmarks in Table 1) before adopting an official policy that human life begins 14 days after fertilization, at a time called gastrulation, when the primitive streak, (the embryonic precursor to the central nervous system) appears. The reason for selecting this time was that following gastrulation the spontaneous division of the blastocyst was not possible, such as might occur when identical twins are formed (also known as twinning). The embryo, after gastrulation, could be unequivocally termed an individual, and not a twin.[17, 39]

Although, we disagree with this particular milestone in light of the evidence we will present, the Warnock Committee's attempt to actively and honestly define a milestone based on science was refreshing. This is in unfortunate comparison to the U.S. Supreme Court's legal abandonment of a more clearly defined, evidence-based scientific consensus regarding abortion.

> **The Warnock Committee adopted a policy that human life begins at 14 days after fertilization, a time called gastrulation.**

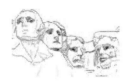

In America

Abortion is not a new issue in America. From Colonial times to the early Republic years, following centuries of common law practice in England and Europe, abortion was permitted as a matter of public health in America. This was seen as an attempt to prevent the loss of the valuable lives of a limited supply of women, who could be injured when trying to obtain illegal abortions.

In 1821, Connecticut enacted the first abortion laws, where abortions of a non-quickened fetus were often permitted. This more lenient approach was generally allowed in order to save the life of the mother.[17]

> **Connecticut in 1821 enacted the first abortion laws—abortions of non-quickened fetuses were treated more leniently than quickened ones.**

In 1973 the U.S. Supreme Court finally ruled on abortion, but it sidestepped the question of when life begins. Justice Blackmun, a former Mayo Clinic Board of Trustees member and counsel, wrote the majority opinion for the Court. He is said to have spent endless hours in the vast Mayo library during the deliberations, and before the ruling, and to have consulted many Mayo medical experts.[18, 40]

Ultimately, though, neither he nor the Court were able to scientifically or philosophically define when life begins. While the Court confessed that it could not define when human life began, the result of the Roe vs. Wade decision was the legal opinion that life comes into being at the point of viability, when the fetus can survive outside the mother's womb. The ruling also arbitrarily prevented states from restricting abortion before the end of the first trimester (12 weeks). The Roe vs. Wade decision implied viability to be from 24 to 28 weeks, based on the medical data available in 1973. And the ruling added that after 12 weeks, abortion should be allowed if the pregnancy endangers the mother's life or health, including her emotional health.[15, 18, 37, 40]

> **While the Supreme Court declared that it could not define when human life began, the result of the Roe vs. Wade decision was the legal opinion that life comes into being at the point of fetal viability.**

The United States' administration, courts, and scientific community, in contrast to the United Kingdom, still does not have any official consensus definition of when human life begins. This lack of a clear definition hinders attempts at legal, ethical, and practical decisions. Unfortunately, emotions, agendas, economics, and politics are usually the primary motivating factors behind these decisions, rather than science and ethics.

The U.S. Supreme Court arbitrarily prevented states from restricting abortion before the end of the first trimester (12 weeks), and that after 12 weeks, abortion must be allowed if the pregnancy endangers the mother's life or health, including her emotional health.

Most historical and contemporary abortion laws in the U.S. originate from a rather vague ability of the ruling agency to define life based upon: popular opinion that life begins at conception; or maybe at quickening; or maybe the viability of the fetus outside the womb; or possibly at birth. To permit the continuation of this ambiguous approach impedes the progress of our scientific community and our society as a whole—it is no longer acceptable.

The United States' administration, courts, and scientific community, in contrast to the United Kingdom, still does not have any official consensus definition of when human life begins.

Figure 1: Female Reproductive Organ

Diagram of the female reproductive anatomy demonstrating the egg in the ovary and then fertilization with the sperm. The fertilized oocyte then travels down the fallopian tube until implantation on day 8.

Female Reproductive Organ

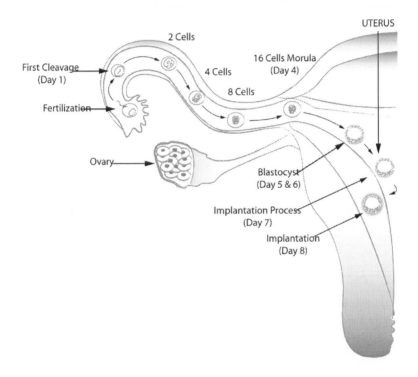

Chapter 4

The Biology of Life's Beginning

In order to understand the basis for the debates about the beginning of human life, we must first review the biology of human reproduction.

Every cell in our body contains our genes on structures called *chromosomes*. Chromosomes are made up of very tight coils of our DNA. *Deoxyribonucleic acid* (DNA) is the material that contains the instructions for each cell in our body to perform its normal function. The DNA in each cell is contained in the nucleus of the cell. Each strand of DNA is divided up into sections, like the sentences in this book—each with a beginning and an end. Each of these "sentences" is called a *gene*, and each gene will provide the instructions to make a specific protein. Each protein has a specific function—one of tens of thousands of metabolic functions—within the cell that allows the cell to function, or "live." Each of the estimated 75 trillion cells in every human being contains about 22,000 pairs of genes—as we inherit one copy of each gene from our mother and one copy from our father. We have one copy of each gene on each chromosome, so that there are on average nearly 1,000 genes on each chromosome. Humans have 46 chromosomes, or 23 pairs. Chromosome pairs 1-22 are called autosomes. The 23rd pair is the sex chromosomes—an X and a Y chromosome. Females have two X chromosomes. Males have one X and one Y chromosome.

Mitosis

Mitosis is the most common form of cell reproduction. This non-sexual type of cellular division simply creates two identical cells (*daughter cells*) from the original cell (*parent cell*). This form of reproduction is similar in every animal. In mitosis, a cell will first replicate the DNA in its nucleus. It then goes through a specific four-stage process where its DNA is first duplicated and then it is divided into two identical copies, followed by a symmetrical division of the remaining cell—resulting in two identical daughter cells with identical sets of DNA. While genetic errors can occur during this process, each new daughter cell will have the same DNA and same set of genes as the original parent cell.

Meiosis

The initial stages of sexual reproduction begin with the establishment of reproductive germ cell lines. Sexual reproduction involves a process known as *meiosis*. Meiosis is the process in which a cell duplicates and then divides its DNA into four daughter cells with each daughter cell containing only one half of the original number of genes.

Table 2: Human Cells Reproduction Terminology	
Mitosis	Classical Cellular Reproduction
Meiosis	Sexual Cellular Reproduction
Human Cells	46 Chromosomes
Daughter cells	½ number of chromosomes (23)
Autosomal Chromosomes	Humans - 22 pair
Sex Chromosomes	Humans - 2 X or 1 X and 1 Y
Zygote	"Tethered together," the unified egg and sperm
Morula	"Mulberry" 16 cells enters the uterine cavity
Early Blastocyst	Contains a cyst or blastocele that develops within the cell mass
Mature Blastocyst	Contains an inner cell mass that becomes the future embryo
Implanted Blastocyst	The blastocyst and inner cell mass that have come into contact with blood from uterine capillaries
Embryo	Implantation to 8 weeks
Fetus	8 weeks

It is important to note that in mitosis, each resulting daughter cell contains a full set of 46 chromosomes. Each of these new cells is a fully capable and functional cell and can perform the same functions as the original parent cell. In meiosis, however, each resulting daughter cell will have only 23 chromosomes. This is only one half of the amount of DNA needed for normal cellular functions, so these cells only have limited capabilities and purpose.

In the female, these four daughter cells are known as primary and secondary *oocytes*. Only one of the four daughter cells will develop into an egg cell, with the other three cells being lost and never used in reproduction. In the male, all four of the daughter cells become four identical *spermatids*. These four cells each then mature so that hundreds of thousands of fully functional sperm cells are eventually created.

Sexual reproduction is the biological process for reproduction in humans and animals. The process results in a fusion of the egg and sperm at fertilization into a single cell. The female egg cell has been stored since before that woman's birth, until one day when it may be released from the ovary—becoming a unique and very special target. It may then be involved in a fusion with one of the millions of sperm cells. This is fertilization, and usually occurs in the *ampulla* of the *fallopian tube*. Fertilization is called conception in humans.[35, 36, 45]

Conception, however, is not a singular event, but a process. Conception involves the penetration of the sperm through the outer layers of egg cell, the oocyte. The fusion of the sperm and oocyte membrane then occurs. This process involves a multitude of cellular and biological arrangements in the membrane at the *cytoplasmic* and nuclear levels.[53, 60]

The oocyte (egg cell)—which amazingly has been paused midway through the second part of meiosis since before that female was born—then proceeds to complete the second part of its meiotic cycle. The result is then a restoration of the full number of chromosomes (46). At this point, the sex of the future individual has been determined.

Conception is not a singular event, but a process.

From here onward, the fertilized oocyte is called a *zygote* (Greek: *tethered-together*). This is the result of the combination of the egg and the sperm. The zygote has a unique complement of DNA and its gender has been determined, but this union in humans is only the beginning of a unique journey (Figures 1 and 2, and Table 2).

On the first day, the zygote begins to divide as it travels down the fallopian tube towards the uterus. The new single cell soon divides through the normal mitotic process, and continuous new divisions occur about every 20 hours. When there are sixteen cells, the zygote is called a *morula* (meaning *mulberry*). The morula leaves the fallopian tube and enters the uterine cavity by the fourth day. Cell division continues and eventually a cavity known as a *blastocele* then forms within the center of the morula.

Individual cells of the morula now begin to flatten. They become more compact on the inside of the cavity. The developing embryo is now called a *blastocyst* (Figure 2, Table 2). Two types of cells now form: the inner cell mass (a cluster of cells together on the inside surface of one side of the blastocele cavity) and the *trophoblast* (the cells lining the sphere of the blastocyst). The inner cell mass is what will become the future embryo.

On the sixth day, the blastocyst begins the process of attaching to the uterine wall. Prior to this point, the uterus has gone through a series of changes in response to a maternal hormone, progesterone. The *uterine endometrial epithelium* (the inner lining of the uterus) has undergone changes in preparation to become a potential site for implantation of the blastocyst. As the blastocyst approaches, the implantation site quickly becomes swollen with new blood vessels called *capillaries*. These vessels and their surrounding cells form the *decidua,* which will further develop and eventually become a major part of the placenta during pregnancy. As the trophoblasts along the side of the blastocyst with the inner cell mass begin to selectively attach to the uterine wall, this initiates a process called *implantation.*

By the seventh day, the blastocyst has invaded the endometrial epithelium of the uterus. Small blastocyst-trophoblast cavities develop to receive the mother's blood. Both the mother's uterus and the blastocyst-trophoblast are simultaneously and rapidly preparing for this important step. The mother's blood will now begin to nourish the new embryo.

By the eighth day, the mother's blood has accessed the embryo and has begun to provide nutrients and oxygen. The established circulation is also clearing the toxic byproducts of the increasingly complex metabolism of the growing number of cells. Blood flow—life's unique mechanism—has been established, providing oxygen and nutrients while clearing out carbon dioxide and other metabolic toxins.

Many developmental benchmarks occur over the next few weeks and months: gastrulation, first heartbeat, neurulation, a recognizable body shape, first brain waves, quickening, and fetal viability. All of these are fascinating and very necessary steps in growth and development, but all are only secondary events that follow implantation. No benchmark surpasses the seminal event of implantation, and the unique contact and subsequent nourishment with a mother's life-giving blood, which occurs on days seven and eight.[49, 58, 59]

Throughout the process of mitosis and meiosis, there may arise many different abnormalities in the number of chromosomes, or in the portions of the chromosomes, being deleted, duplicated, or altered. These mishaps may result in unbalanced numbers of chromosomes or genes in the daughter cells. A fusion of one of these abnormal egg or sperm cells at conception may result in chromosome or other genetic abnormalities. Some of these abnormalities may not be compatible with life and miscarriages may then naturally occur. Other abnormalities may still be able to result in a living person, but these individuals may have a range of genetic disorders.

> **By the 8th day, the close contact between the growing blastocyst and the endometrial uterine lining has been established and fulfills a vital step for the new embryo.**

It is not known how often fertilization continues to a successful pregnancy. Defective zygotes with genetic abnormalities are not uncommon. They most commonly are lost within the first few weeks of a pregnancy, some not even recognized, passing through as regular, or slightly delayed, menstruation. Some research has estimated that up to 68% of conceptions may be lost during the first trimester of pregnancy.[61] A normally conceived and delivered human baby may, in fact, be a minority of zygote formations.

> **The many milestones are fascinating and necessary steps in growth and development, but none surpass the seminal event of implantation.**

Additional genetic concerns have to also be considered. One powerful factor in development—genetic imprinting—involves another layer of complexity beyond even these very intricate cellular and chromosomal divisions and duplications that have already occurred.

Imprinting

While the Human Genome Project resulted in complete DNA sequences for humans and many other organisms, it did not fully reveal how we control the expression of our genes. We have found that our genes are turned on or off by many inherited and environmental factors at specific times by mechanisms that we are only now discovering, and by other mechanisms that we have yet to discover.

Epigenetics is the study of the modifications and factors influencing gene expression that are not encoded through our DNA sequence. This inherited system is coupled to, and set upon, the DNA received from our parents and results in turning each gene on or off in specific places and times.

These epigenetic controls are dependent upon a form of genetic regulation called *methylation*—where specific genes can be "methylated." Methylation refers to the addition of a methyl group to the DNA nucleotide cytosine (or less commonly adenine). When genes are methylated, the methylated genes are inactivated and cannot be expressed. Those specific genes cannot then make the specific protein that has a specific designated function. In contrast, a gene that is not methylated will quickly make a specific protein, which then produces its specific metabolic cellular function. At any time, thousands of genes are active (non-methylated), while thousands of others are inactive (methylated).

Genetic imprinting is the phenomenon controlling how genes inherited from the mother and father are expressed in different ways. There are significant events in genomic imprinting that continue during the development of the early zygote. When the Human Genome Project was

38

proposed, and then successfully completed, many of us had hopes that a full understanding of human life would now be at our fingertips. Though, alas, we in biology and science should not have been so naïve. Science and biology are always deeper and more complex than we initially imagine.

> **When the early zygote cells divide, they maintain their own energy needs—there is no external nourishment.**

Imprinting and methylation is a complex process unique for each sperm and egg prior to fertilization. The sequence of how genes are turned on at certain times while others are turned off is very specific. This is essential to each individual cell's unique growth and development into hundreds of differentiated cell and tissue types at specific locations and times throughout embryonic development—and throughout the entire life of the individual.

Methylation is an extremely complex inherited process. It provides the driving force of our genome with precision tuning. Specific imprinting is essential to normal development of the growing embryo. Imprinting abnormalities lead to developmental failures as early as the two cell stage—occurring minutes to hours following fertilization.[62] The genomes of the sperm and egg are both inactive at the time of fertilization due to imprinting.[63] It is not until the blastocyst stage, around day eight post-fertilization, and immediately prior to or during implantation, that signs of new methylation specific to the future embryo appear.[63]

The imprinting process following conception suggests that biologically, the genetic identity of a new life is not determined until near day eight post-fertilization, at the time when the blastocyst has developed and implantation is occurring.

> **At the blastocyst stage, around the eighth day post-fertilization and during implantation, there are new signs of methylation specific to the future embryo.**

This review of embryologic development and genetics has to be compared with the current opinions on when human life begins. We have seen there is a continuous process where the sperm and egg are specifically formed,

39

and then come together at conception. This is the earliest point at which there is a complete set of DNA. All 46 chromosomes are present. However, this new genome is not active—and does not become active—until around the eighth day after fertilization. Prior to that time, the cells divide while maintaining their own energy needs—as there is no external nourishment for the zygote as it becomes two cells, then four cells, then eight cells, and then the sixteen cell morula. As the morula enters the uterine cavity, it only then begins to turn into the blastocyst containing the inner-cell mass and the surrounding outer cells that will then become the future placenta.

There is no specific or unique time point that would differentiate the zygote-morula-blastocyst as a unique individual.[64]

> **The imprinting process following fertilization suggests that biologically, the genetic identity of a new life is not determined until around the eighth day after fertilization, interestingly, at the same time that the blastocyst has implanted and the mother's blood is beginning to nourish a new life.**

Genetic Identity

The popular argument is that the completion of all 46 chromosomes represents the earliest moment of a unique individual, with a unique genetic identity. That argument can no longer accurately be defended, given what we now understand about genomic imprinting.

There are also many other aspects we should consider. Such factors include the already cited evidence of a very high spontaneous miscarriage rate during these first few days. Many zygotes do not reach the blastocyst stage, and many more fail to implant and pass through with the next menses.

In addition, there is the inactivation of either the paternal and/or the maternal halves of the new genome—until about the eighth day post-fertilization. This important fact tells us that these cells do not yet compose a new genetic individual. While the morula will have specific sex

40

chromosomes to determine the future sex of the individual, these cells do not have a specific gender, nor are the newly combined maternal and paternal "halves" of DNA functionally active. While sexual identity is a simple measure of individuality, there is obviously a great deal more involved with the expression of thousands of different genes. Many other individual determinates are also not set until that same time point—when the blastocyst begins implantation.

Fertilization is the earliest point when there is a complete set of DNA. All 46 chromosomes are present, but this new genome is not active and does not become active until around the eighth day post-fertilization due to methylation processes.

Blastocyst Viability—and Implantation

Another popular misunderstanding that necessitates some comment centers on the question of blastocyst viability. The blastocyst is the earliest stage from which new life can begin. In the laboratory, an artificially fertilized egg *in vitro* can develop into a zygote and then a morula. And while it may have the genome to become a new life, it can never become a human life without first becoming a blastocyst. Even then it must be implanted in a mother's uterus. Otherwise it will die and disintegrate on its own, just as the uterus will not support the blastocyst if it is not precisely prepared at that exact time.

The zygote-morula-blastocyst contains limited energy reserve—just enough to get it to the implantation time. In vitro fertilization clinics and stem cell research labs will preserve cell lines by quickly freezing them. Without freezing or implanting, the blastocyst withers and disintegrates. The next natural step—implantation—marks the critical step in the developmental process. The in vitro blastocyst has three paths: natural disintegration, frozen status, or implantation. While cells may be taken out of the central cell mass for stem cell research (such as cloning), even these cells—which could be cultured into new zygotes, or morula, or blastocysts—will face the same ultimate fate: natural disintegration, frozen status, or implantation. No new fetus, baby, or person can be brought forth without eventual implantation into a mother's uterus to be nourished by her blood.

From a scientific, biological, and genetic viewpoint, this thesis would support the real beginning of human life as being on the eighth day, shortly after implantation and contact with a mother's blood. However, in secular science—divorced from moral, ethical and religious aspects—the question may actually be moot—as secular science does not desire to engage these aspects in its deliberations. It is not moot in reality, since we live in a complex world, full of good and evil that cannot be reduced to simple chemistry, physics, or biology. For those who accept only a secular worldview, we submit that the best scientific, biological, and genetic marker for the beginning of human life is directly after implantation—when a mother's blood begins to nourish the otherwise doomed blastocyst.[58, 59]

For those who choose to look to, and accept, a higher authority to help guide their ethics and actions, we now proceed beyond politics, history, biology, and genetics.

> **There is inactivation of either the paternal and/or the maternal halves of the new genome—until the eighth day post-fertilization. Thus these cells are not yet a new genetic individual and his/her future identity is not determined until a later time point—the eighth day.**

Figure 2: The Three Parts of a Blastocyst

The Three Parts of a Blastocyst

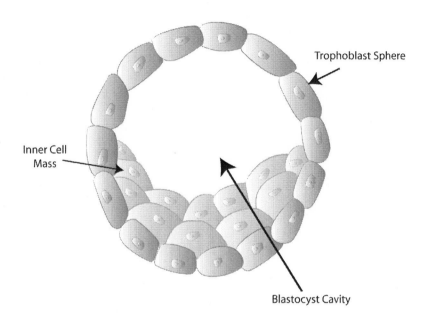

Chapter 5

The Biblical Evidence:
The Breath of Life & Life in the Womb

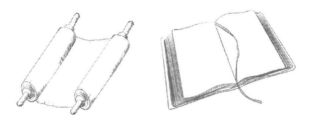

The moral and ethical question indeed is—when does an individual human life begin? The populist view has been at conception—the time of the union of the sperm and the egg (i.e. fertilization). As we have seen in earlier chapters, this view has been based upon philosophy, Greek logic, ecclesiastical edits, historical decisions, and political considerations—but is this view supported by the current understandings of embryonic development as here documented? The answer is no. In fact, the modern biological and genetic evidence presented in the previous chapter reveals that human life begins, not at a "moment" of conception, but at implantation on the eighth day, when contact with maternal blood occurs. This coincides with important changes in genetic expression due to imprinting that also occur on day eight.

So, is this compelling information from cutting edge biology the final determinate? If there were nothing else, as it is said in Hebrew, "Dayanu – It would be enough." But we should not stop there, lest in fact, there be more. Beyond biology, can we find more evidence supporting a focus on this time point? Is there a moral basis? Do the scriptures support, or contradict, the biology and genetics of when human life begins? [6]

This chapter gives an overview of this scriptural evidence, providing a summary sufficient to fully understand the thesis, and enough detail for a compelling case to be made (with future information forthcoming at www.LifeBeginsWhen.org).

Much has often been inferred about the beginning of life stemming from the scriptures used in the Christian, Jewish, and Islamic faiths. All three faiths share a common foundation of teachings derived from the writings of the book of Genesis.

In the lengthy writings and discussions of "When does human life begin?" it is surprising and unfortunate that the Genesis record of the creation of man is often missed, ignored, or quickly passed over.

Such examples include the discussions by the Presidential Council on Bioethics. These scholarly and well-thought works are worth reading and reflect current philosophical, ethical, and political dialogues, but are an example of our point: The biblical account in the book of Genesis is not considered. Again, in the Christian deliberations spanning St. Augustine to Pope Pius IX, there is a loud absence of discourse regarding the creation of Adam in the book of Genesis. With that in mind, we will not make the same oversight. In fact, we will start with this Genesis record as a foundation, fully understanding what is said there before investigating the many other relevant biblical records.

> **There is NO scripture which states that human life begins at conception.**

First we must make it clear that, despite the many prevailing assumptions, there are absolutely no scriptures stating that human life begins at conception. Our thorough search of scriptures in English, Hebrew and Greek, exhaustive searches of hundreds of theological volumes, commentaries and lexicons, and our challenge to many biblical scholar friends and associates, have found no such definitive biblical declaration.

There are, however, inferences (discussed in detail later this chapter) that address a level of individual awareness in utero—implying life is present in the mother's womb. We concur with this implication, but not with the conclusion that intra uterine life means life starts at conception.

Bear with us through this chapter. Although an understanding of the biblical basis of "When does human life begin?" is simple, it cannot become clear without seeing all the evidence and understanding the whole picture, as presented in the scriptures.

Let's be crystal clear. We should initially focus our attention on the singular and most momentous event of when the first man first drew the breath of life. This designates the origin of humanity, according to the Bible. And this is often overlooked. This event, where the *breath of life* is given to Adam, marks a clear defining moment—the beginning of a specific human life. Beyond this, the Bible contains many more references emphasizing the connection between life and the presence of breath.

Breath of Life

The earliest biblical reference to the beginning of human life is found in Genesis 2:7:

> "And the LORD God formed man of the dust of the ground, and breathed into his nostrils the *breath of life*; and man became a *living soul*." [emphasis added]

Here is an important link: the breath of life and a living soul. Genesis 2:7 reveals an entirely new concept about how life begins. This is a completely new way of thinking, not found among the other ancient societies and religions. This relationship is also often forgotten in our modern world.

In order for man to become a "living soul" (Hebrew: *nephesh chaya*), God breathed (Hebrew: *naphach*) into his nostrils the "breath of life" (Hebrew: *neshmat chayim*). The Hebrew words reveal much about this tight relationship and important foundation.[67, 68, 69]

The Hebrew words for "soul" and "breath" have the same root—*nephesh*. Man becomes a "living soul" because he has the "breath of life."

Table 3: Hebrew root word relationships:	
Neshma / Neshmat	Breath
Naphach	Breath, "Breathe out"
Nephesh	Soul
Ruach	Wind, Breath
Chai / Chaya / Chayim	Life, Living

Neshmat chayim literally means "breath of life." In this phrase, *neshmat* cannot stand alone, and is linked to *chayim* (life).

Putting the Hebrew terms into the English text of Genesis 2:7 powerfully reinforces this relationship:

> "And the LORD God formed man of the dust of the ground, and *naphach* (breathed) into his nostrils the *neshmat chayim* (*breath of life)*; and man became a *nephesh chaya* (*living soul).* "

It should be noted that man did not obtain a soul, nor does he "have" a soul. Rather he *became* a soul, specifically, a *living* soul. This theological concept is quite profound, but currently outside the scope of this thesis, other than to emphasize that the man is, with the breath of life, a living soul. It is not within the concept of the lexical and contextual meaning of "soul" to separate out a distinct essence. The soul is the essence of the living man. That is what he is, and he is so, because he has the breath of life in him.

There is another Hebrew word, *ruach*. It is most often translated as "wind", "breath" or "spirit". *Ruach* is often used interchangeably with *nishama*, the word from which we get *neshmat* in Genesis 2:7. As we examine other verses using *ruach* and *neshmat*, we can clearly see that it is the "spirit" or "breath" of God that gives life unto his creation. Two of the numerous biblical examples are listed here:

> "The *Spirit* (*Ruach*) of God has made me, and the *breath* (*neshmat*) of the Almighty gives me *life* (*chayim*)." (Job 33:4)

> "...and the *breath* (*ruach*) came unto them; and they *lived* (*chayu*)." (Ezekiel 37:10)

These and numerous associated passages clearly link obtaining the breath of life with the start of becoming a *nephesh chaya*, a living soul. So when the breath of life is lost, does that then represent death? From among the numerous references to this, we will illustrate two examples:

> "I will bring a flood…to destroy all life wherein is the *breath of life* (*ruach chayim*)." (Genesis 6:17)

> "All in whose nostrils was the *breath of the spirit of life*…died (*neshmat ruach chayim*)." (Genesis 7:22)

This breath-life relationship is not limited to the Tanach (Old Testament). New Testament scriptures are preserved in the Greek language and the Greek root words mirror their Hebraic roots. They reflect the same Hebrew ideas, but in the Greek language.[77,78]

Greek terms, like their Hebrew counterparts, associate breath and life with a breathing, living, soul.

The Greek word *psuche* is similar to the Hebrew *nephesh*, meaning "soul," or a "breathing being." The Greek *pneuma* is like the Hebrew *neshama* and *ruach*, and also means "breath," "wind," and "spirit." *Zoe*, the Greek word for "life," is analogous to the Hebrew *chai*. These Greek terms, like their Hebrew counterparts, associate breath and life with a breathing, living soul. Some examples of this usage can be seen in Acts 17:24-25, I Corinthians 15:45, James 2:26, and Revelation 16:3.

Now, the Hebrew terms *ruach* and *neshmat* (wind, air, breath, spirit) and the Greek *pneuma* (wind, air, breath, spirit) are certainly used in spiritual, mystical, and allegorical terminology for bigger spiritual lessons. But if their physical reality is not understood, their idiomatic and midrashic applications would be voided. We will discuss these in later volumes.

The point at this time should be clear: a human life begins with the breath of life, and ends with loss of the breath of life.

Having established this important link between life and breath, we must consider a logical question that then immediately comes to mind:

Does human life begin at the first breath of air at birth?

From the evidence presented so far, concluding that life begins at birth, with the first breath would seem a logical biblical position. After having confirmed this association between breath and life, one could conclude that life begins when the fetus emerges from the womb and takes its first breath of air. Some prominent and influential Christian and Jewish scholars have indeed taken this position, based primarily on the evidence we have presented so far. But others have doubt.[22, 28, 29, 71, 72, 73, 74]

There is, in fact, a great deal more still to consider. We have a foundation, but not yet all the evidence. Using scripture as a basis for moral and ethical decisions, there are additional important references that we should not ignore.

Life in The Womb ... in Utero

There are many scriptural references to individuals already in existence as unique personalities while in the womb, before breathing their first breath. These individuals are described as having already achieved a state of personhood, and a personhood of special value. We must take into account these many scriptures that picture an individual life as already in existence in utero (in the womb). These references would be *non sequitur* if a human life—a living soul—began at one's first breath (i.e. at birth).

Among these thought-provoking scriptures is the famous example relating to the Hebrew prophet Jeremiah, who was described as being set-apart and sanctified in utero:

> "The word of the LORD came unto me, saying; Before I formed you in the belly I knew you; and before you came forth out of the womb I sanctified you, and I ordained you a prophet unto the nations." (Jeremiah 1:4-5)

This reference is famous, as it is often considered a primary biblical proof-text for human life beginning at conception. Although this verse does not specifically say that God recognized Jeremiah as an individual at conception, it clearly does state that God knew Jeremiah as a special individual, with an anointed destiny, before he was born—while he was in the womb. It could even be extrapolated back to a time before he had human form, very early in the gestational process.

Some insight can be extracted from the Hebrew text. The Hebrew word used for "formed" here in Jeremiah 1 is not from the well known Hebrew root of *bara'* ("create"), nor from the Hebrew root of *asah* ("made"). Rather it is an infrequently used Hebrew word, *etzor*. This Hebrew term, instead of referring to creating or making, refers directly to an act of sculpturing—like in pottery. It pictures something being shaped into a literal physical form.[68] This verse, if read literally (although one needs to take care in doing so in poetic settings), extends the individual personhood of Jeremiah back to before he had a recognizable human form, to a very early time in his mother's uterus. Either way, whether read as literal or poetic, this scriptural allegory provides a firm witness for life in utero. This time point clearly predates later time points, such as viability and birth. It does not point to the exact time of his personhood, however. Any of the first fifteen milestones listed in Table 1 could fit. (The reader may already understand which milestone is a best fit.)

Another illustration is a very melancholic and dark poem, a depressing description by the prophet Jeremiah at one stage of his prophetic service. Here he is lamenting why and how he was alive to suffer so much, and why was he not killed while he was in his mother's womb. Why did the womb not become his grave?

> "Because did he not kill me in the womb, so my mother would have been my grave, and her womb forever great. Why did I come out from the womb, to see toil and sorrow, and spend my days in shame?" (Jeremiah 20:17)

This sorrowful poetry similarly describes Jeremiah as being alive in his mother's womb. His apparent wish that the womb would become his grave, were he to die in utero, suggests life in the womb. Not answering his question, but keeping our purpose and focus here, he is clearly implying that he was already alive while in the womb.

Several other prophets are described as existing, and receiving special callings from God, in utero. The prophet Isaiah was called from within his mother's womb:

> "Listen, O isles, unto me; and hearken, you people, from far; The LORD has called me from the womb; from the bowels (belly) of my mother has he made mention of my name." (Isaiah 49:1)

Like Jeremiah, Isaiah paints a word picture of himself as having personal identity and purpose before his birth, even while gestating in his mother's womb. These are not the only persons so described in scripture.

The account of Job, in the book bearing his name, is a deeply philosophical and ethical drama; a work that is considered to be among the most ancient of scriptural texts. Here, Job, after a long series of tragedies, reflects on his state of affairs. He describes himself as living in the womb. Then he ponders what would have become of him should he have died in utero, or passed out without being noticed.

> "Why did you bring me out from the womb? Would that I had died before any eye had seen me and were as though I had not been, carried from the womb to the grave." (Job 10:18-19)

Samson, the famous biblical strongman, is another example. He was dedicated as a Nazarite while in his mother's womb. His mother kept the strict Nazarite purification rites for his sake, although he was not yet born. (Judges 13:7; 16:17)

These scriptural references to individual human life existing in the uterus, before birth, are not limited to the Hebrew Scriptures.

The New Testament, reflecting its Hebrew background, relates to an event where Mary, carrying Jesus in her womb, met with her cousin, Elizabeth, who was pregnant with John the Baptist. The record states that Elizabeth's unborn child, the prophet John, leaped in utero when Elizabeth heard of Mary's good news, that she was pregnant with Jesus. Elizabeth was about in her sixth month of pregnancy.

> "And it came to pass, that, when Elizabeth heard the salutation of Mary, the babe (John) leaped in her womb." (Luke 1:41)

These examples clearly illustrate the biblical notion that individual life already exists during pregnancy, before birth.

The initial evidence seemed to point to human life being closely associated with the ability of an individual to actually breathe in the *breath of life*. However, this is contrasted with those prophets who were all described as distinctive human beings—individuals with special callings and individualized responses before birth, in utero, prior to delivery from the mother's womb.

> **Many scriptures describe various prophets as unique, living individuals while in the womb, including Jeremiah, Isaiah, Job, Samson, and John.**

So how can we reconcile these two separate concepts? How can we explain the apparent existence of human life in utero—*before* they took their first breath, the *breath of life*?

Were these people merely implied to be alive, or were they actually considered living individuals? Is their individuality merely an expression of their unique genetic identity, their potential to ultimately become the person they were destined to become, or is there some other explanation?

> **How can we reconcile these two separate concepts of 1.) life in utero with 2.) the taking of a first breath— the *breath of life*?**

The next array of scriptural evidence is, we propose, a key that is well known to both scriptural scholars and laypeople, but which, to the authors' knowledge, is lacking coverage in the hundreds of articles and scores of volumes exploring this subject. When understood, it explains the puzzle and presents a unified and truly beautiful picture of *when human life begins*.

Chapter 6

Blood … The Key

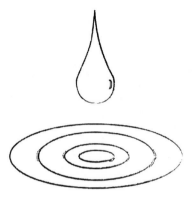

Throughout the Bible, there is great importance attached to the blood of a being—whether human or animal. Sacrifices have been a part of human culture in all societies, in all areas of the earth, in every time, up until the modern world. In fact, they remain a part of many cultures today. These sacrifices were usually animal, but some were human. Although this is a somewhat foreign concept to the modern mind, scientists still speak of "sacrificing experimental animals" or even "sacrificing embryos." The term is so much a part of our language that it spills over into baseball in the "sacrifice fly." But sacrifice in the ancient world was not taken lightly, and it almost always included a blood ritual.

The scriptures not only recognize blood sacrifice, but also command such through a system of elaborate blood rituals. Early in the book of Genesis, we have Adam and Eve covered with skins of animals—implying animals had to die for them to be covered. The first sons, Cain and Abel, are pictured offering sacrifices, and even here we actually begin to see the importance of blood. Abel's blood sacrifice was accepted, but the vegetable sacrifice from Cain was not. All the patriarchs from Noah to Abraham and down to Moses worshipped the Creator with the shedding of animal blood. The Torah itself can be seen as containing a set of elaborate ceremonies for Israel, which from the very beginning, were tied to the tabernacle and later the temple. Scholars correctly call this system a blood cult.

The importance of blood in scripture is not limited to animal sacrifices. Reverence for blood, animal or human, was instilled into the culture. When an animal was killed for meat, its blood was to be drained and covered with dirt. Anyone with an "issue" of blood—from wounds, injury, menstruation, childbirth, disease, etc.—was to avoid public assemblies in order to maintain pure and sanitary societal conditions.

Finally, there was prohibition against eating (or drinking) blood. Although animal flesh was eatable (after the blood was drained), the Tanach (Old Testament) placed a special emphasis on the blood of an animal. Here are the distinct prohibitions against eating or drinking blood:

> "You shall not eat flesh with its life, that is, its blood."
> (Genesis 9:4)

> "And if anyone of the house of Israel or of the strangers who sojourn among them eats any blood, I will set my face against that person who eats blood and will cut him off from among his people." (Leviticus 17:10)

> "Be sure that you eat not the blood ..." (Deuteronomy 12:23)

These blood rituals and their importance did not end with the destruction of the Jewish temple in 70 C.E. In fact, blood continued as a central theme of New Testament and Christian doctrine. The shed blood of Jesus on the cross, the "eating of his flesh, and drinking his blood" at the Christian Lord's Supper, or Eucharist, is central to Christian practice. Even animal sacrifice still continues within Islam.

It is interesting that the prohibition against eating blood, given through Moses, did not cease in Apostolic times. These warnings against the consumption of blood continued into the New Testament and the early church period. In the book of Acts, Jesus' disciples, now the Apostles, were soon challenged after his death, resurrection and ascension, with what to do with the flood of proselytes and Gentiles joining their ranks. After considerable deliberation, the Jerusalem Council in Acts 15 established certain requirements that new converts must follow within the growing church.

"For it seemed good to the Holy Spirit, and to us, to lay upon you no greater burden than these necessary things: that you abstain from things offered to idols, from blood, from things strangled." (Acts 15:28-29)

It is rather interesting to see that of all the possible issues and doctrines that could have been highlighted, that the prevention of eating blood—as those things strangled would contain un-drained blood—was among these. Why was there such a strict code against ingesting the blood of an animal? Why was this a central issue and conclusion in the early Christian congregations? Statements from Deuteronomy and Leviticus clarify this:

"Only be sure that you eat not the blood, for the blood is the *life* (*nephesh*); and you may not eat the *life with the meat*." (Deuteronomy 12:23)

"For the *life* (*nephesh*) of the flesh is in the blood: and I have given it to you upon the altar to make atonement for your souls; for it is the blood that makes atonement for the soul." (Leviticus 17:11)

The scriptural reason given for not consuming blood is that the life of the animal is in the blood! This is further highlighted in other scriptures such as in Genesis 9:4, Leviticus 17:11, and Deuteronomy 12:23. This prohibition against eating blood is an example of its importance. It is indicative of the central role that blood plays in Hebrew and Christian worship, morality, and theology.

We will not review all the well-known biblical references to blood at this time, in order to allow the reader to quickly get to our primary point. We will, however, briefly highlight some of the numerous links and associated themes of the Old and New Testaments regarding the importance of blood:

- When an animal was sacrificed, its blood was spilled and its life came to an end.
- The blood ritual was the heart of the Old Testament sacrificial system.
- The "shedding of blood" is a metaphor for losing one's life or being killed.
- Blood is central to the Passover and Exodus from Egypt.

- The personal and corporate atonement of the people and nation of Israel could not be achieved without the shedding of blood.
- The Messiah's blood atonement is central to New Testament theology.
- The Messiah's blood atonement is central to The Crucifixion.
- The Eucharist has associations with the significance of the Messiah's shed blood.

Much more can and will be said about this point in the future, and can be easily referenced by anyone with a Bible (see also www.LifeBeginsWhen.org).

The association of breath and life should be well understood at this point. But now we see an additional association with life—blood, leading us to a point of seeing that life is associated with breath, and with blood. Indeed, even the Brown-Driver-Briggs Hebrew and English Lexicon[68] confirms that the term *nephesh* is clearly linked with both "breath" and "blood." It says *nephesh* with *chai* is specifically "a living being whose life resides in the blood."

Blood: The Missing Link in Life's First Breath

From scriptural evidence, we have seen in earlier chapters that human life first appears to begin with the *breath of life*—which many may initially presume is at the first breath of air. Additional evidence then demonstrated that life actually exists earlier in the womb before birth. However, there is a gap between these times (a nine month period in utero vs. the specific moment of birth) as laid out in the biblical account. In trying to unite the common elements of these points, one must search for a unifying theme. This has naturally led to many proposals regarding various milestones in human embryonic development, such as the presence of a heartbeat, or a nervous system, or the form and movement of an individual person (See Table 1).

Upon this debate then, we add a new layer, when we understand that life ends when the *breath of life* is lost with the shedding of blood.

We propose, based on the science laid out in chapter 4, and the scriptural definition of life in chapters 5 and 6, that it is the presence of blood as the element that remains common in all of these descriptions.

Blood—carrying the breath—is what defines the beginning and end of life. Life's first breath is not the presence of air in the lungs, but the presence of a mother's blood to provide the vital elements (nutrition and oxygen) for life (Hebrew: *nephesh chaya*) to begin.

The most commonly held view today among traditional, non-modernist Christian communities is that human life begins at conception. This is based solely on an outdated understanding of human physiology and genetics. That view of human life beginning at conception, presents an inconsistency with scripture, with the necessity of blood being a vital element for life. At conception, there is no breath of life provided by blood, as blood does not nourish the zygote or blastocyst before implantation.

Now, we should pause a moment to consider what blood is. Blood is one of our many organ systems. The study of blood in medicine is called hematology, and includes diseases of the blood. Blood is a very complex liquid tissue, composed of many dozens of cell types, hundreds of chemicals and hormones, and thousands of proteins types. These all derive from thousands of different genes from both the mother and father and are unique to each individual. There are hundreds of functions for the blood. It has a multifaceted ability to deliver nutrients essential and unique to each of our diverse tissues, while meeting the common needs of every tissue with a supply of oxygen and the ability to remove carbon dioxide, toxins, and accumulations of organic acids. It is essential to our immune responses and it has complex clotting mechanisms to seal off breaks in blood vessels.

The largest component of the blood is the erythrocytes—red blood cells. They make up 40-50% of our blood's volume. These cells are filled with hemoglobin. Hemoglobin captures oxygen molecules as it passes through the vessels of the lung. Each hemoglobin molecule can carry four oxygen molecules. These are delivered to the various body parts, enabling them to function in an oxygen-enriched environment. Hemoglobin carries so much oxygen that over 98% of the body's oxygen is at any one time attached to hemoglobin. Other body fluids (without hemoglobin) contain less than 2%. So, of the many thousands of functions of blood, the most critical at any and every moment is the delivery of vital oxygen by hemoglobin to the various tissues.

We see then that blood maintains a central role in human and animal physiology. So it should not be unexpected that human life is linked to blood. Consequently, we should not be surprised that in scripture there is also a central role of blood in identifying a human life. This link, we propose, is the critical link in understanding when human life begins.

This is why we point to the time of implantation of the blastocyst as the focal point for the beginning of human life.

Some have objected to the concept of a *nephesh chaya*—a living soul—being defined by the circulation of blood, despite the clear and often repeated emphasis of blood in the scripture. Some have claimed there is sufficient oxygen in the fallopian tube before implantation supplying the zygote indirectly.

This may seem to be a compelling contra-argument, but is it true? It is a fact that there is oxygen all around us: in the air, in the soil, in the water, and in our tissues. However, if those levels were sufficient for human and animal life, we would need no lungs, no heart, no circulatory system, and no blood. All tissues could receive vital oxygen by diffusion.

This would further ignore the facts of biology. Oxygen content is measured in units called PaO_2—the partial pressure of oxygen. It is usually expressed as a percent saturation. The air around us, what we breathe, is 20%. Our bodily fluids, other than blood, are about 5%. The arterial blood—coming from the heart and circulating through our lungs—is nearly 100%. In other words, it is super-saturated. It is four to five times the concentration of oxygen in the atmosphere. It is designed and primed to deliver an abundant load of oxygen to our many body tissues. This allows each of these tissues to be able to perform their highly active and metabolically demanding functions such as growth, repair, movement, thought, vision, hearing, etc. Of interest, our brain may require nearly 25% of the oxygen needs of the entire body. Without this abundant, super-saturated source of oxygen, our brain ceases to function and will encounter severe damage within five minutes—as is commonly seen in those who have suffered a stroke, heart attack, or were the victim of drowning. Our muscles, heart, liver, and other tissues may be able to survive for a few minutes longer, but even those tissues have only limited time. This happens to all our cellular processes that are highly oxygen dependent.

In biology, we say that the cells that require abundant oxygen are dependent on aerobic glycolysis. They need high levels of oxygen to perform their very active metabolic processes. Conversely, there are some cells in our body that do not always require the same dependence on oxygen for their metabolic function. They are able to temporarily function using anaerobic glycolysis. Anaerobic glycolysis is the process of deriving energy from sugar and other nutrients, without oxygen. For instance, muscle cells are able to perform both aerobic and anaerobic glycolysis. This is seen when a marathon runner runs at a rather slow pace for 3-4 hours, and can run over 26 miles before exhausting his energy stores. This pace allows aerobic glycolysis (burning sugar via oxygen dependent processes) to deliver the energy needed. In contrast, a sprinter can run all-out and cover 100 yards in less than 10 seconds—at speeds many times a marathon runner, but he cannot sustain this intense energy requirement without oxygen for more than a few hundred yards. This is possible only because he is temporarily producing energy for the muscles from quick release anaerobic glycolysis. These chemical stores are burned up quickly, and he must rest before they can be restored and he can run again. The anaerobic glycolysis comes from limited energy reserves that are not oxygen dependent.

So what does this have to do with the beginning of human life? We know that the zygote following the fusion of the egg and sperm is developing through various stages to become the blastocyst over a seven-day period. This is an extremely long time on a cellular level. The egg has developed and stored enormous stores of energy in order to be able to complete this seven-day journey following fertilization. It also is going through mitosis as it divides, but the overall cell mass does not increase. Its store of energy is limited to only a few days requirements. These energy stores are overwhelmingly anaerobic.[79, 80, 81, 82, 83, 84, 85,91] This means it is utilizing glucose by converting it to pyruvate and lactate as it develops into a blastocyst without oxygen—anaerobically.

By the 8th day, the maturing blastocyst has utilized almost all its anaerobic energy stores. If the zygote, after having now become a blastocyst, does not rapidly implant, its anaerobic energy stores will soon be totally depleted. It will disintegrate within the next two to three days. The zygote—starting with the fusion of the sperm and egg—develops within a setting of low oxygen partial pressure. In fact, the partial pressure of the fluid in the fallopian tube and uterine cavity is much less even than atmospheric levels. [79, 80, 86,91]

If the blastocyst has been able to implant, it will thrive and rapidly develop in the oxygen rich environment provided by the mother's blood. The rapidly developing embryo is highly dependent on receiving this life sustaining oxygen-rich blood.[86] We are all aware of the dire consequences of any disruption of this vital blood flow from the mother through the placenta to the fetus later during pregnancy. Implantation is the vital initial step to begin this dependence upon the blood—the breath of life. Without this step, the zygote-blastocyst development will stop and life will not occur.

Medical teams that grow fertilized zygotes for artificial insemination and transfer for infertile couples, keep the zygote cultures at an oxygen percentage of only 5%. They keep the cultures in a high nitrogen and low oxygen environment. [87, 88, 89, 90] High oxygen levels (even the 20% in our atmosphere) will cause stress to the zygote and prevent its development. All of this is explained in detail so we can be clear about the centrality of implantation with its delivery of highly oxygenated blood. This highly oxygenated blood is the source of the "breath of life" that marks the beginning of a *nephesh chaya*—a living soul and an individual with the full personhood—with all the respect due a living soul. For all of his/her life span, it is this life-giving blood that sustains every individual person.

We should now point out that here we are discussing the life of an individual human being, whose individual life is sustained by the blood. The same terminology can and is applied to animals in the scriptures. However, we must distinguish a *nephesh chaya* from "cellular life." Other forms of life such as bacteria, fungi, coral, jellyfish, and plants are living single-celled or multi-celled forms of life. These other forms of living things fill our planet's air, water, and ground. They are inside of and even cover our bodies. These cellular life forms thrive in settings with just atmospheric oxygen concentrations, and some in locations with little or no oxygen. To some oxygen is even toxic, but none of these other life forms needs the oxygen nourishment of blood, and are not *nephesh chaya*—living souls. The biological term "life" certainly applies to them. For the sake of this discussion, we focus upon the biblical definition of a living soul—*nephesh chaya*—which is limited to those living creatures, including man, whose life is sustained by the blood (see Brown-Driver-Briggs Hebrew and English Lexicon).[68]

In the next chapter we will summarize how scripture and biology agree that life begins immediately after the implantation of the embryo into a mother's uterus. That is the time when a mother's blood begins to supply the breath of life, the life-giving and life-supporting nutrition, oxygen, and environment to create a *nefesh chai*, a "living soul" with the "breath of life."

This occurs on or about the eighth day after conception.[58, 59]

Chapter 7

A Compelling Case for Implantation

Human life begins at implantation—not at birth, not at conception, not at viability, and not at 40 days. This perspective provides a fresh approach—not in that it is unknown or even new,[76] only that it is so often overlooked, and yet it is so straightforward, so simple, and so logical. More importantly, though, is that this position provides a solution which is founded upon a solid scientific understanding of reproduction, genetics and embryology, and that is consistent with scripture. We don't fault the ancients and medieval scholars for what they could not have known, but today in the 21st century it is time to acknowledge the information that scientific and medical advancements have made available. The blinds are off!

For those on the pro-abortion side, you are challenged to a respectful discussion and evidence-based debate. For those on the pro-life side who look to scripture, we as physicians and scientists join you and honor you in our mutual love of life. We agree that abortion is an unwarranted destruction of life (*nephesh chaya*), but life is not destroyed until after implantation. That is the time contact is made with the mother's life-giving blood that carries essential nourishments (including oxygen, the *breath of life*) to the embryo and giving it life (*nephesh chaya*). This occurs on day seven or eight.

The key problem with the U.S. Supreme Court's 1973 decision was related to misunderstandings and a lack of consensus as to when human life begins. Justice Blackmun studied the subject for nine months in the same library and institution where the authors have trained and collectively spent 25 years. Justice Blackmun and his Court decided to rest their decision on traditions, guesses, and ultimately, political compromises. The result has been more extreme polarization, more confusion, and accelerating conflicts. This confusion has spilled over into issues of contraception and stem cell research (that did not exist in 1973).

This book is an introduction into our many years of work and research, beginning long before the stem cell and in vitro fertilization research and applications further raised the debate—and amplified the rhetoric. We believe the Court's previous inability to find a scientific, historical, and religious answer cannot now be sustained in view of this fresh evidence.

Our thesis separates the abortion question from the contraception and stem cell research debates. These issues often cloud, and even dilute, the case against abortion. This was not the purpose of the study, but a consequence. The appeal of preserving a "living soul" (*nephesh chaya*), based on scientific and scriptural evidence should provide the pro-life position with a much clearer and more compelling voice. Most importantly though, we submit it provides clarity from a scientific and scriptural basis for a new evidence-based consensus.

Our conclusion is that a human egg and human sperm union cannot become a *nephesh chaya* ("living soul") without implantation into the uterus, which then provides nourishment from a mother's blood—carrying the *breath of life*.

Even an in vitro artificially fertilized egg, zygote, or morula can never become a human life without first becoming a blastocyst AND THEN being implanted into a uterus. It is emphasized that for in vitro fertilized and cloned embryos, as well as for naturally conceived zygotes, implantation is the seminal event—and the best point to mark the beginning of human life.

We reiterate: all future embryos must reach the blastocyst stage and must then be implanted into the uterus, where the mother's blood feeds it the breath of life (oxygen) in order to become a human life.

We point out that:

- A human embryo cannot grow outside of a uterus via a placenta.
- No human being (nor any animal) can be grown in a test-tube or biotic chamber. There is no such thing as a test-tube baby.
- No in vitro fertilization or even cloning products can become a human life without implantation.

- Cloning, whether of sheep, cattle, primates or humans, are not births from a test tube. They all proceeded through implantation of the blastocyst, and are born only from a uterus.

Finally, we need to mention cells harvested from the central cell mass of the blastocyst before implantation. These cells, which have never come into contact with blood and its life-giving "breath," can indeed grow in tissue cultures into individual muscle, nerve, or bone tissues, etc. They can produce up to 220 different kinds of human tissues. This is, of course, the hope of stem cell research—a hope millions of people anticipate. These wonderful cells cannot, however, become new individual human beings (*nephesh chaya*) without implantation into a uterus.

Table 1 lists 23 milestones in developmental biology, and individual and social development, which have been proposed throughout history as time points where one could have confidence declaring: "This is when human life begins." Conception, gastrulation, heartbeat, brain waves, quickening, viability and birth have been leading viable contenders for various reasons (to be discussed in later editions and on our web site). However, to date, none have produced that "ring of truth" or presented compelling evidence from scientific, moral and scriptural foundations.

The authors present this work for consideration to all who would like a fresh approach—an approach for those who would choose to form their ideas, beliefs and practices not upon assumption, dogma, tradition, or emotion, but on the solid evidence of history, science, and scripture.

We conclude that human life begins within hours of the implantation of a blastocyst into the uterine *mucosa*.

This is the time:

- When there is a massive burst of biochemical and cellular events
- When most imprinting—methylation—has peaked
- When the inner cell mass of the blastocyst begins to receive the essential nutrients, including oxygen, from a mother's blood
- When a mother's blood can clear away toxic metabolic waste products
- When the blastocyst has truly become an embryo, in the classical sense

- When this new embryo is receiving the breath of life from a mother's blood

This is the time—when a new life—*a nephesh chaya* begins.

Notes and References:

1. Daniel Oliver, "Deciding Abortion, The Key Questions," *National Review* 57, no. 8 (2005): 25–26.

2. Louis M. Guenin, "Stem Cells, Cloning and Regulation," *Mayo Clinic Proceedings* 80 (2005): 241–250.

3. Louis M. Guenin, "A Proposed Stem Cell Research Policy," *Stem Cells* 23 (2005): 1023–1027.

4. Louis M. Guenin, "The Nonindividuation Argument Against Zygotic Personhood," *Philosophy* 81 (2006): 463–503.

5. Bernard Williams, "Types of Moral Argument Against Embryo Research," in *The Ciba Foundation Symposium* (1986): 185–212.

6. G. Khushf, "Owning Up to our Agendas: The Role & Limits of Science in Debates about Embryos and Brain Death," *Symposium: Defining the Beginning and the End of Human Life: Journal of Law, Medicine & Ethics* (Spring 2006): 58–76.

7. Peter Singer, *Unsanctifying Human Life,* ed. Helag Kuhse (Blackwell, UK: Oxford Press, 2002).

8. Gary Rosenkrantz, "What is Life?" ed. In Tian Yu Cao, *Proceedings of the Twentieth World Congress of Philosophy* 10 (2001): 125–134.

9. Bernard Williams, *Ethics and the Limits of Philosophy* (Cambridge, MA: Harvard University Press, 1995).

10. Jack Wilson, Biological Individuality, The Identity and Persistence of Living Entities (Cambridge, UK: Cambridge University Press, 1999).

11. Richard Arneson, "What, If Anything, Renders All Humans Morally Equal?" in *Singer and His Critics*, ed.

Dale Jamieson (Blackwell, UK: Oxford University Press, 1999), 103–128.

12. Norman M. Ford, *When Did I Begin?* (Cambridge, UK: Cambridge University Press, 1988).

13. Helga Kuhse and Peter Singer, "Individuals, Humans and Persons: The Issue of Moral Status," in *Embryo Experimentation*, ed. Peter Singer, et al. (Cambridge, UK: Cambridge University Press, 1990), 65–75.

14. Francis J. Beckwith, "Defending Abortion Philosophically: A Review-Essay of David Boonin's 'A Defense of Abortion'," *Journal of Medicine and Philosophy* no. 31 (2006)

15. Roe v. Wade, 410 U.S. 113 (1973). (Argued December 13, 1971. Reargued October 11, 1972. Decided January 22, 1971.).

16. James Witherspoon, "Reexamining Roe: Nineteenth-Century Abortion Statutes and the Fourteenth Amendment," *St. Mary's Law Journal* no. 17 (1985): 29–77.

17. Laurence H. Tribe, *Abortion: The Clash of the Absolutes* (New York, NY: W.W. Norton & Company, 1990).

18. Francis J. Beckwith, "The Supreme Court, Row vs. Wade, and Abortion Law," Liberty University Law Review 1 no. 1 (2006).

19. Plato, "Phaedo" in *The Republic and Other Works*, trans. Benjamin Jowett (New York, NY: Anchor Books, 1973), 498.

20. G. Bonner, "Abortion and Early Christian Thought," in *Abortion and the Sanctity of Human Life*, ed. J.H. Channer (Exeter, UK: The Paternoster Press, 1985), 93–122.

21. D. DeMarco, "The Roman Catholic Church and Abortion: A Historical Perspective," *The Homiletic and Pastoral Review* (July 1984): 59–66.

22. Jakobovits, "Jewish Views on Abortion," in *Abortion Society and Law*, ed. D. Walbert and J. Butler (Cleveland, OH and London, UK: The Press of Case Western Reserve University, 1973), 103–121.

23. H. J. Morowitz and J.S. Trefil, *The Facts of Life: Science and the Abortion Controversy* (New York, NY: Oxford University Press, 1992).

24. M. Buss, "The Beginning of Human Life as an Ethical Problem," *Journal of Religion* no. 47 (1967): 244–255.

25. Tertullian, *Apology* 9:7-8, eds. Alexander Roberts and James Donaldson, trans. The Ante-Nicene Fathers (Grand Rapids, MI: Eerdmans Publishing, 1994).

26. D. DeMarco, "The Roman Catholic Church and Abortion: A Historical Perspective," *The Homiletic and Pastoral Review* (July 1984): 59–66.

27. Aristotle, *History of Animals* Book VII, Chapter 3, 583b.

28. L. Zoloth, "The Ethics of the Eighth Day: Jewish Bioethics and Research on Human Embryonic Stem Cells," in *The Human Embryonic Stem Cell Debate: Science, Ethics, and Public Policy*, ed. Suzanne Holland, Karen Lebacqz and Laurie Zoloth (Cambridge, MA: MIT Press, 2001).

29. Tohoroth II Oholoth 7:6, *Talmud* (as cited by Jakobovits 1973).

30. Thomas Aquinas, *Summa Theologiae* Vol 6, II, 50, trans. Ceslaus Velecky, Timothy Suttor and Colman E. O'Neill (Cambridge UK: Cambridge University Press, 2006).

31. Aaron L. Mackler, *Introduction to Jewish and Catholic Bioethics, A Comparative Analysis* (Washington, D.C.: Georgetown University Press, 2003).

32. D. Marquis, "Why Abortion is Immoral," *The Journal of Philosophy* no. 86 (1989): 183–202.

33. John Haldane and Patrick Lee, "Aquinas on Human Ensoulment, Abortion and the Value of Life," *Philosophy* no. 78 (2003): 255–278

34. Pius IX, "Apostolicae Sedis Moderationi," in *Acta Apostolicae Sedis* 5 (1869): 305–331.

35. Scott F. Gilbert, Anna L. Tyler and Emily J. Zackin, *Bioethics and the New Embryology, Springboards for Debate* (Sunderland, MA: Sinauer Associates, Inc. and

Gordonsville, VA: W.H. Freeman & Company, 2005), 31–45.

36. Scott F. Gilbert, "Bioethics: When Does Human Life Begin?" in *DevBio, A Companion to Developmental Biology*, 2003, Seventh edition, http://www.devbio.com/article.php?id=162/.

37. H. J. Morowitz and J.S. Trefil, *The Facts of Life: Science and the Abortion Controversy* (New York, NY: Oxford University Press, 1992).

38. D. A. Jones, "The Human Embryo in the Christian Tradition: A Reconsideration," *Journal of Medical Ethics* no. 31 (2005): 710–714.

39. Eugene Mills, "Dividing Without Reducing: Bodily Fission and Personal Identity," *Mind* no. 102 (1993): 37–51.

40. Joseph W. Dellapenna, "Abortion and the Law: Blackmun's Distortion of the Historical Record," in *Abortion and the Constitution: Reversing Roe vs. Wade Through the Courts*, ed. Dennis J. Horan, Edward R. Grant and Paige C. Cunningham (Washington, DC: Georgetown University Press, 1987), 137–158.

41. Woosuk Park, "The Problem of the Individuation for Scotus: A Principle of Indivisibility or a Principle of Distinction?" *Franciscan Studies* no. 48 (1988): 105–123.

42. Dennis J. Horan and Thomas J. Balch, "Roe vs. Wade: No Justification in History, Law, or Logic," in *Abortion and the Constitution* (1987): 57–88.

43. R.M. Sade, "Introduction: Defining the Beginning and the End of Human Life: Implications for Ethics, Policy, and the Law," *Symposium: Defining the Beginning and the End of Human Life: Journal of Law, Medicine & Ethics* (Spring 2006): 6–7.

44. M. Tooley, "Abortion and Infantcide," in *Bioethics: An Anthology*, ed. H. Kuhse and P. Singer (Oxford, UK: Blackwell Publishers, 1999).

45. Scott F. Gilbert, *Developmental Biology*, 2006, 8th edition.

46. T.W. Sadler, *Langman's Medical Embryology*, 9th ed. (Baltimore, MD: Lippincott, Williams and Wilkins, 2004).

47. William Larsen, *Human Embryology*, 3rd ed. (Philadelphia, PA: Churchill Livingstone, 2001).

48. Ronan O'Rahilly and Fabiola Muller, *Human Embryology and Teratology* (New York, NY: Wiley-Liss, 2001).

49. M. B. Renfree, "Implantation and Placentation," in *Reproduction in Mammals 2: Embryonic and Fetal Development*, ed. C.R. Austin and R.V. Short, 2nd ed. (Cambridge, UK: Cambridge University Press, 1982), 26–69.

50. Peter R. Brinsden, A Textbook of In Vitro Fertilization and Assisted Reproduction, The Bourn Hall Guide to Clinical and Laboratory Practice, 2nd ed. (New York, NY: Parthenon Publishing, 1999).

51. M. B. Renfree, "Implantation and Placentation," in *Reproduction in Mammals 2: Embryonic and Fetal Development*, ed. C.R. Austin and R.V. Short, 2nd ed. (Cambridge, UK: Cambridge University Press, 1982), 26–69.

52. Joseph F. Donceel, S.J., "Immediate Animation and Delayed Hominization," *Theological Studies* 31 (1970): 76–105.

53. Philip G. Peters, Jr., "The Ambiguous Meaning of Human Conception," *UC Davis Law Review* no 40 (2006): 199ff.

54. N.M. Ford, When Did I Begin? Conception of the Human Individual in History (New York, NY: Cambridge University Press, 1988).

55. Thomas Shannon and Allan B. Wolter, "Reflections on the Moral Status of the Pre-Embryo," *Theological Studies* 51 (1990).

56. B. Steinbock, Life Before Birth: The Moral and Legal Status of Embryos and Fetuses (New York, NY: Oxford University Press, 1992).

57. *Donum Vitae* (Vatican City: The Holy See, 1987): quoted in *Infertility: A Crossroad of Faith, Medicine, and Technology*, ed. Kevin W. Wilkes (The Netherlands: Kluwer Academic Publishers, 1997), 209–238.

58. J.L. Merritt, J.L. Merritt II and B.P. Merritt, "The Beginning of Human Life: The Central Role of Implantation in Developmental Biology and Historical Records," *Ethics Section, International Society for Stem Cell Research,* Barcelona, Spain (July 9, 2009).

59. J.L. Merritt, J.L. Merritt II and B.P. Merritt, "Historical and Biological Reviews: The Role of Implantation and Life's Beginning," *Ethics Section, World Stem Cell Summit 2008*, Madison, WI (September 22, 2008).

60. Fazale Rana, *The Cell's Design* (Grand Rapids, MI: Baker Books, 2008).

61. O. Francis, "An Analysis of 1150 Cases of Abortions from the Government R.S.R.M. Lying-In Hospital, Madras," *J Obstet Gynaecol India* 10 no. 1 (September 1959): 62–70.

62. W. Shi and T. Haaf, "Aberrant Methylation Patterns at the Two-Cell Stage as an Indicator of Early Development Failure," *Molecular Reproduction & Development* 63 no. 3 (November 2002): 329–334.

63. A.L. Kierszenbaum, "Genomic Imprinting and Epigenetic Reprogramming: Unearthing the Garden of Forking Paths," *Molecular Reproduction & Development* 63 no. 3 (November 2002): 269-272.

64. R. Templeton, "When Does Life Begin?" in *The Embryo: Scientific Discovery and Medical Ethics*, ed. S. Blazer and E.Z. Zimmer (Basel, Switzerland: S Karger AG Publishers, 2005), 1–20.

65. Sacred Congregation for the Doctrine of the Faith, *Declaration on Abortion* (Vatican City: The Holy See, 1974): reprinted in *Vatican Council II: More Postconciliar Documents* vol. 2 (Collegeville, MN: The Liturgical Press, 1982), 441–453.

66. Louis M. Guenin, *The Morality of Embryo Use* (Cambridge, UK: Cambridge University Press, 2008).

67. *New English Bible* (Wheaton, IL: Crossway Bibles, 2008).

68. F. Brown, S. Driver, and C. Briggs, *The Brown-Driver-Briggs Hebrew and English Lexicon* (Peabody, MA: Hendrickson Publishers, 1999), 659, 675.

69. *BibleWorks 8.0* DVD-ROM (Virginia Beach, VA: BibleWorks LLC, 2009).

70. William D. Mounce, *The Analytical Lexicon to The Greek New Testament* (Grand Rapids, MI: Zondervan Publishing House, 1993), 233, 379, 487.

71. J. Woolf, I. Kennedy, R. Deech and L. Donaldson, *Law, Medicine and Ethics: Essays in Honour of Lord Jakobovits*, ed. Freilich Carrier and Parbhoo Joffbrand (London: The Cancerkin Center, Royal Free Hospital, 2007).

72. J.M. Cohen, Dear Chief Rabbi, from the Correspondence of Chief Rabbi Immanuel Jakobovits on Matter of Jewish Law, Ethics and Contemporary Issues 1980-1990 (Hoboken, NJ: KTAV Publishing House, Inc., 1995).

73. I. Jakobovits, Jewish Medical Ethics, A Comparative and Historical Study of the Jewish Religious Attitude to Medicine and Its Practice (New York, NY: Block Publishing Company, 1959).

74. "Defining the Beginning and the End of Human Life: Implications for Ethics, Policy and Law," presented at the *Thomas A. Pitts Memorial Lectureship*, Medical University of South Carolina (September 10–11, 2004).

75. J. H. Kurtz, *Offerings, Sacrifices and Worship in the Old Testament*, trans. James Martin (Peabody, MA: Hendrickson Publishers, Inc., 1998).

76. Orrin Hatch, *Square Peg: Confessions of a Citizen-Senator* (New York, NY: Basic Books, 2002.), 229–242.

77. W.F. Arndt, F.W. Gingrich, A Greek-English Lexicon of the New Testament and Other Early Christian Literature (Chicago, IL: The University of Chicago Press, 1957.) 340-342, 680-685, 901-902.

78. J.P. Louw, E.A. Nida, Greek-English Lexicon of the New Testament Based on Semantic Domains, 2nd ed (New York, NY: United Bible Societies, 1989, in Logos Bible Software 4, 2010.)

79. P. Guerin, S.E. Mouatassim, Y. Menezo. "Oxidative stress and protection against reactive oxygen species in the pre-

implantation embryo and its surroundings." *Hum Reprod Update* 2001;7:175– 189.

80. L. Mastroianni Jr, R. Jones, "Oxygen tension within the rabbit fallopian tube." *J Reprod Fertil,* vol 147, 1965, 99 –102.

81. D.K. Gardner, H.J. Leese, "Concentrations of nutrients in mouse oviduct fluid and their effects on embryo development and metabolism in vitro," *J. Reprod Fertil,* vol 88, 1990, 361-368.

82. M. Lane, D.K. Gardner, "Lactate regulates pyruvate uptake and metabolism in the preimplantation mouse embryo," *Biology and Reproduction,* vol 62, 2000, 16-22.

83. M. Lane, D.K. Gardner, "Mitochondrial malate-aspartate shuttle regulates mouse embryo nutrient consumption," *J. Biological Chemistry*, vol 280, 2005, 18361-18367.

84. A. Jurisicova, S. Varmuza, R.F. Casper, "Programmed cell death and human embryo fragmentation," *Mol Hum Reprod* , vol 2: 1996, 93-98.

85. Z. Wiener-Megnazi, L. Vardi, A. Lissak, S. Shnizer, A.Z. Reznick, D. Ishai, et al, "Oxidative stress indices in follicular fluid as measured by the thermochemiluminescence assay correlate with outcome parameters in in vitro fertilization," *Fertility and Sterility,* vol 82 (Suppl 3), 2004,1171-1176.

86. D. Sakkas, J.D. Vassalli, "The preimplantation embryo: development and experimental manipulation," *Reproductive Health*, http://www.gfmer.ch/Books/Reproductive_health/The_prei mplantation_embryo_Development_and_experimental_ma nipulation.html

87. T. Paszkowski, A.I. Traub, S.Y. Robinson, D. McMaster, "Selenium dependent glutathione peroxidase activity in human follicular fluid." *Clin Chim Acta,* vol 236, 1995,173-180.

88. J. Cohen, A. Gilligan, W. Esposito, T. Schimmel, B. Dale, "Ambient air and its potential effects on conception in vitro," *Hum Reprod*, vol 12, 1997, 1742–1749.

89. A. Agarwal, T.M. Said, M.A. Bedaiwy, J. Banerjee, J.G. Alverez, "Oxidative Stress in an Assisted Reproductive Techniques Setting," *Fertility and Sterility*, vol 86; 3, Sept 2006, 503-512.

90. A.J. Watson, P.H. Watson, D. Warnes, S.K. Walker, D.T. Armstrong, R.F. Seamark, "Preimplantation development of in vitro-matured and in vitro-fertilized ovine zygotes: comparison between coculture on oviduct epithelial cell monolayers and culture under low oxygen atmosphere," *Biol Reprod,* vol 50, 1994, 715-724.

91. J.L. Merritt, J.L. Merritt II, "Zygote to blastocyst development prior to implantation is not oxygen dependent," 2011, World Stem Cell Summit, Pasadena, CA, 2011.

Additional Resources

www.WhenDoesHumanLifeBegin.com

www.CrystalClearBooks.org